Antipsychotics

The Story of a Drug

Painkillers: History, Science, and Issues
Victor B. Stolberg

Antipsychotics

HISTORY, SCIENCE, AND ISSUES

Jeffrey Kerner and Bridget McCoy

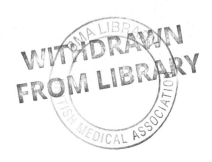

The Story of a Drug
Peter L. Myers, Series Editor

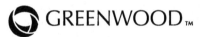

GREENWOOD™

An Imprint of ABC-CLIO, LLC
Santa Barbara, California • Denver, Colorado

Library of Congress Cataloging-in-Publication Data

Names: Kerner, Jeffrey, author. | McCoy, Bridget, author.
Title: Antipsychotics : history, science, and issues / Jeffrey Kerner and Bridget McCoy.
Description: Santa Barbara, California : Greenwood, an Imprint of ABC-CLIO, LLC, [2017] | Series: The story of a drug | Includes bibliographical references and index.
Identifiers: LCCN 2016042476 (print) | LCCN 2016043096 (ebook) | ISBN 9781440839887 (hardcopy : alk. paper) | ISBN 9781440839894 (ebook)
Subjects: LCSH: Antipsychotic drugs. | Antipsychotic drugs—History. | Psychoses—Chemotherapy.
Classification: LCC RM333.5 .K47 2017 (print) | LCC RM333.5 (ebook) | DDC 615.7/882—dc23
LC record available at https://lccn.loc.gov/2016042476

ISBN: 978–1–4408–3988–7
EISBN: 978–1–4408–3989–4

21 20 19 18 17   1 2 3 4 5

This book is also available as an eBook.

Greenwood
An Imprint of ABC-CLIO, LLC

ABC-CLIO, LLC
130 Cremona Drive, P.O. Box 1911
Santa Barbara, California 93116-1911
www.abc-clio.com

This book is printed on acid-free paper ∞

Manufactured in the United States of America

Contents

Series Foreword   *ix*
Acknowledgments   *xi*
Introduction   *xiii*

Chapter 1: Case Studies   **1**
Case 1: Jimmy   1
Case 2: Bobby   7
Case 3: George   14

Chapter 2: What Are Antipsychotics?   **19**
Psychotic Disorders and the Symptoms of Psychosis   19
Treatment of Psychosis: From Exorcism to Antipsychotics   25
Typical Antipsychotics: The Beginning   28
Atypical Antipsychotics: As the Story Continues. . .   42

Chapter 3: Antipsychotics: A Brief History   **51**
Early Biologic Remedies: The Original Antipsychotics   53
"A Drug in Search of an Illness": Developing Antipsychotic
Medications   57
Chlorpromazine Rises   60
Side Effects Emerge   64
Competition for Chlorpromazine   65
How Antipsychotics Are Used Today: Bridging Past and Future   69

Chapter 4: How Antipsychotics Work   73
Parts of the Brain   74
What Are Neurotransmitters and What Do They Do?   76
Neurotransmitters Affected by Antipsychotics   77
Other Potential Targets   91

Chapter 5: Effects and Applications   93
Therapeutic Effects of Antipsychotics   93
How Well Do Antipsychotics Work?   103
Indications for Medical Use   107
Antipsychotic Use in Special Groups   117

Chapter 6: Risks, Misuse, and Overdose   123
Side Effects   123
Misuse of Antipsychotics   147
Antipsychotic Overdose and Toxicity   148

Chapter 7: Production, Distribution, and Regulation   151
Pharmaceutical Industry   151
Antipsychotics in Nursing Homes   159
Prior Authorization   160
The Unique Case of Clozapine   161
AIMS and Metabolic Monitoring   165

Chapter 8: The Social Dimensions of Antipsychotics   169
Deinstitutionalization   170
Antipsychotics and the Doctor-Patient Relationship   174
Legal and Ethical Implications of Antipsychotics   178
Antipsychotics and Political Dissent   184
Antipsychotics and the Elderly   185
Antipsychotics and Children   186
When to Treat? The Implications of the Initiation of Antipsychotic
Treatment   188
The Business of Antipsychotics   189
Mental Illness and Violence   190

Chapter 9: The Future of Antipsychotics   193
Where Are Antipsychotics Failing?   194
Pathophysiology of Chronic Psychotic Disorders   198
New Medications on the Horizon   200

Better Routes of Administration   205
Use in Nonpsychotic Disorders   211

Directory of Resources   *217*
Glossary   *221*
Bibliography   *227*
Index   *231*

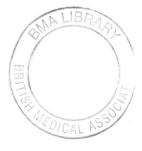

Series Foreword

While many books have been written about the prevalence and perils of recreational drug use, what about the wide variety of chemicals Americans ingest to help them heal or to cope with mental and physical issues? These therapeutic drugs—whether prescription or over-the-counter (OTC), generic or brand-name—play a critical role in both the U.S. health-care system and American society at large. This series explores major classes of such drugs, examining them from a variety of perspectives, including scientific, medical, economic, legal, and cultural.

For the sake of clarity and consistency, each book in this series follows the same format.

We begin with a fictional case study bringing to life the significance of this particular class of drug. Chapter 2 provides an overview of the class as a whole, including discussion of different subtypes as well as basic information about the conditions such drugs are meant to treat. The history and evolution of these drugs are discussed in Chapter 3. Chapter 4 explores how the drugs work in the body at a cellular level, while Chapter 5 examines the large-scale impacts of such substances on the body and how such effects can be beneficial in different situations. Dangers such as side effects, drug interactions, misuse, abuse, and overdose are highlighted in Chapter 6. Chapter 7 focuses on how this particular class of drugs is produced, distributed, and regulated by state and federal governments. Chapter 8 addresses professional and popular attitudes and beliefs about the drug as well as representations of such drugs and their users in the media. We wrap up with a consideration of the drug's possible future, including emerging controversies and trends in research and use, in Chapter 9. Each volume in this series also includes a glossary of terms and a collection of print and electronic resources for additional information and further study.

It is our hope that the books in this series will not only provide valuable information but will also spur discussion and debate about these drugs and the many issues that surround them. For instance, are antibiotics being overprescribed, leading to the development of drug-resistant bacteria? Should antipsychotics, usually used to treat serious mental illnesses such as schizophrenia and bipolar disorder, be used to render inmates and elderly individuals with dementia more docile? Do schools have the right to mandate vaccination for their students, against the wishes of some parents?

As a final caveat, we wish to emphasize that the information we present in these books is no substitute for consultation with a licensed health-care professional, and we do not claim to provide medical advice or guidance.

—Peter L. Myers, PhD
Emeritus member, National Addiction Studies Accreditation Commission
Past president, International Coalition for Addiction Studies Education
Editor-in-Chief Emeritus, *Journal of Ethnicity in Substance Abuse*

Acknowledgments

I would like to acknowledge the places and people that inspired me to write this book. I wrote this book in a broad variety of locations, and the texture of the physical space in which I wrote is present in the words. I started this book on a fall day at the Wave Hill gardens in the Bronx, overlooking the Hudson River and my native New Jersey. I wrote the section on side effects while I was in prison, so apologies if it comes off as hard and intense. I was not an inmate; I was working as a psychiatrist at Sing Sing Correctional Facility, but, in the literal sense, I did in fact write this section when I was *in* prison. I wrote the rest in my apartment in Riverdale, in various public libraries and cafés, and in the reading room at the Tisch Library at Tufts University, where my medical studies began with inorganic chemistry in 2001.

More importantly, I would like to recognize the people who contributed to this work. I am grateful to my parents, Martin and Susan Kerner, who taught me how to write. I am grateful to the individuals who taught me how to practice psychiatry. I think first about my patients. I know that I have not always been successful in relieving their pain. I hope that I effected as much positive change in their lives as they did in mine. I also thank my teachers and mentors at Montefiore Medical Center, especially Andrea Weiss, MD, Merrill Rotter, MD, and Matthew Schneider, MD.

This book is for Lisa and Charlie, my deepest loves.

Jeffrey Kerner

I would like to acknowledge the people who have helped me along the way to be the person I am today, working on and toward what I am passionate about. That starts with my parents who always supported me and never told me what I should do with my life, but always made me feel like I could do anything. My influential English literature professors in high school and college who helped to instill my fascination and intrigue with the human psyche and understand a person's story. More recently, my teachers and mentors at Montefiore Medical Center who have encouraged my growth as a physician, psychiatrist, and, most importantly, an individual. And finally, my partner, who helps me continue to grow into the person I want to be and challenges me to always be ready to engage with the world through different perspectives. Thank you.

Bridget McCoy

Introduction

Mental illness is a public health concern that touches everyone in one way or another. By some estimates, about 40 percent of the population will be affected with some form of mental illness at some point in their lives. If we include parents, siblings, children, and best friends, it becomes a near statistical certainty that either we ourselves or someone we are extremely close to will suffer from a mental illness. When there is a crisis, we turn to our loved ones long before we find a mental health professional. Therefore, everyone, in a way, is an amateur psychiatrist.

The most prevalent illnesses include problems with depression, anxiety, substance use, and personality disorders. Because of the ubiquitous nature of mental illness, psychiatric medications are commonly prescribed and are now widely accepted. Antidepressants, a class of medications used to treat depression and anxiety, are among the most prescribed class of medications.

This text describes antipsychotics, the class of medications primarily used to treat psychotic illnesses. Broadly speaking, psychosis refers to a break with reality. Psychotic illnesses, like schizophrenia and schizoaffective disorders, have, and continue to be, some of the most challenging illnesses to treat. Physicians have attempted to cure these disorders of the mind for millennia with limited success. Even within the past 100 years, some of the most common and medically accepted treatments have proven to be more dangerous than the illnesses themselves. Furthermore, these therapies generally conferred no benefit to the patient.

Antipsychotics were first developed in the 1950s and have dramatically advanced the treatment of the most serious mental illnesses. They have allowed patients to live dignified lives in the community. Prior to the introduction of antipsychotics, these patients could spend their entire lives in psychiatric institutions, tormented by paranoid delusions, auditory hallucinations, and other debilitating symptoms of psychosis. However, as this book explains at length, antipsychotics are hardly perfect medications. They do not always completely address all symptoms of the mental illness, and they have serious side effects. Responsible psychiatrists use antipsychotics with caution.

This text reviews the different types of antipsychotics, the history of their development, their mechanism of action, their risks and side effects, the business of their production, the social implications, and the future of antipsychotics. We will also provide several case studies of typical patients who would be prescribed antipsychotics. These case studies are based on real patients we have treated. Furthermore, we discuss the practice of prescribing antipsychotics in the real world. We will invite the reader to put themselves in the position of the psychiatrist, weigh the various risks and benefits of treatment, and understand the challenges posed to psychiatrists by both the medications and the illnesses they treat.

While the focus of this text is a class of medications, the more important story is about the people who take antipsychotics. We describe illnesses that require the medications and the challenges posed to patients. It is exceedingly difficult for patients with serious mental illnesses to remain compliant with medications and the broader treatment plan. This is primarily due to the fact that paranoia and difficulty discerning reality from delusion is central to psychotic illness. In order to maintain routine medical treatment for any serious condition, it is critical to form a positive and trusting therapeutic relationship with treatment teams. This is difficult for patients who are more likely to be paranoid of others' motives. Furthermore, disorganization is a prominent symptom of psychotic illnesses, which makes it very difficult for well-intentioned patients to attend appointments consistently and remember to take medications. If these hurdles were not enough, patients with serious mental illness are much more likely to have substance use disorders, serious medical conditions, few financial resources, and limited support in the community.

These colossal challenges facing patients with psychotic illnesses will be a recurring theme in this book. We hope to highlight and elucidate the tough odds faced by patients with serious mental illnesses to encourage and grow the reader's empathy. It is very common for mental health practitioners to become cynical and blame patients for frequent relapses due to noncompliance with medications and substance use. Empathy for patients' struggles is the only antidote for cynicism. Even the most disorganized and psychotic patients retain a keen awareness of doctors' attitudes. If they sense the psychiatrist is dismissive, or even in a rush, there will never be the strong therapeutic alliance necessary for treatment and recovery.

The reader should use this text to gain a robust understanding of antipsychotics' role in mental health treatment. In the recent past, any type of mental illness carried a heavy stigma. People would rarely discuss symptoms, let alone that they were being treated with psychiatric medications. Now, the awareness of anxiety, depression, and antidepressants has increased to the point where people generally feel comfortable openly discussing their experiences. We hope this text contributes to a similar destigmatization of psychotic illness and antipsychotics, so affected individuals can also receive widespread support.

Chapter 1

Case Studies

CASE I: JIMMY

Jimmy grew up with his mom in a nice suburban town in the Northeast. His parents divorced when he was five years old, and his father moved to Florida. Jimmy never really understood why his parents split up, but sometimes his mom referred to his father's "problems." His father usually remembers to send a card for Jimmy's birthday but never leaves a phone number.

Jimmy sometimes got jealous of his other friends who had two parents in the house, but otherwise, he never really thought about it too much. Jimmy and his mom had a great relationship. She worked as a radiology technician in a hospital and usually worked overnight. Jimmy's mom was there after school, she took him to all of his after-school activities, and they always did fun things together on the weekends. Jimmy's mother was a great cook, and they often cooked meals together, including fancy pastries.

Jimmy got along well with his friends until about middle school. He and his friends were no longer interested in the same things. Jimmy's childhood friends spent all of their time playing and talking about sports. Jimmy didn't really care about sports. He was more into science fiction. Jimmy's friends thought he was weird because all he talked about was aliens and spaceships. Eventually they stopped inviting him out. Jimmy's mom got concerned that his childhood friends didn't want to hang out with him anymore, but Jimmy didn't really care. He was perfectly content spending time in his room, reading sci-fi comic books and drawing pictures of creatures from outer space. Jimmy still spent time hanging out with his mom.

Jimmy did well academically, but he didn't quite meet his mother's high standards. She thought he was so bright and had so much potential. She knew he could get straight A's and go to an Ivy League school. As in turned out, Jimmy got mostly B's. When he didn't understand something in class, he got very frustrated and gave up. During the spring of senior year, Jimmy was accepted into the engineering school at State University. He didn't want to go to the prom, but his mom kept bugging him. Finally he agreed to go and took his mom's best friend's daughter, who went to another school about half an hour away. Jimmy thought the whole occasion was awkward and weird.

Jimmy spent most of the summer before college at home. He and his mom took a little road trip to visit his grandparents at their house in the country. Otherwise, he spent most of the time in his room, on his computer, looking at science fiction websites, and watching movies. His mom wished he would socialize more, but he was a good kid who stayed out of trouble and she loved him. When she nagged him about spending more time with friends, he reminded her that he chatted with many friends online. Some of his friends went to school with him, other friends he met through sci-fi forums.

Jimmy was anxious before going to State, but he transitioned well. His mom was sad to see him go but was happy for him. His new roommate seemed nice. For the first weeks of college everything was fine. He was doing well in his classes and started going to events sponsored by the sci-fi interest group at State. After a couple weeks, however, things started to change. Jimmy lost interest in his courses. He stopped going to classes consistently and spent almost all of his time in his room, in bed. His roommate started getting worried about him and also was annoyed by the fact that Jimmy was always in his room and never gave him any privacy. When Jimmy came home for Columbus Day weekend, his mom knew something had changed. She thought that he was depressed but couldn't figure out why. She asked him how his classes were, but he didn't want to talk about it. He just stayed in his room in his pajamas the entire weekend until she drove him back to school.

This pattern continued for the next month, and when Jimmy's mom picked him up for Thanksgiving, his roommate told her that he was *really* concerned. He told her that he stopped going to class completely and stays in the room all day and all night.

Jimmy's mom was terrified. She didn't know how to help Jimmy or what to say to him. During the hour-long car ride back, after she demanded that he tell her what was going on, he started to cry, which his mother had never seen. He spent the entire Thanksgiving break in his room and didn't want to go back to school, but his mom insisted.

Jimmy failed all of his classes, and the dean placed him on an academic leave for a semester. Jimmy's mom was beside herself. She scheduled an appointment for Jimmy to see his pediatrician, but he refused to go. She told the pediatrician what was going on, and a referral was quickly made to a local mental health center. Jimmy refused to go to that appointment too. He just stayed in his room for weeks and weeks.

Soon, Jimmy's behavior began to change again. He seemed worried and looked out of the windows as if someone were watching the house. He barely spoke to his mom, but when he did, he only wanted to discuss the Central Intelligence Agency (CIA) and the National Security Agency (NSA). Jimmy's mom woke up a couple times in the middle of the night because she heard a noise and found Jimmy pacing around the hallways.

One afternoon, she smelled marijuana coming out of his room. She was angry and surprised, because she had never seen Jimmy smoking anything or even drinking alcohol. She asked Jimmy what was going on, but he was acting very strange. He was giggling and muttering incomprehensible things to himself. She attributed some of his bizarre behavior to the marijuana, as she had seen friends use the drug before, but she never saw anyone act like that. She told Jimmy sternly that he was not to use any drugs ever again, and she made another unsuccessful attempt to convince him to speak with a mental health professional.

Soon after, she noticed similarly odd behavior even when Jimmy wasn't smoking marijuana. He started laughing and talking to himself. He repeatedly asked his mom if she had been contacted by the NSA or CIA.

One night, Jimmy's mother was awakened several times by noise coming from Jimmy's room, but she tried to sleep through it. In the morning, she knocked on his door, and there was no answer. She knocked again, and he screamed at her to leave him alone, which was an extremely unusual way for Jimmy to speak to his mother. Jimmy's mom tried to open the door, but something was blocking it. She pushed harder and harder and finally managed to open the door wide enough to fit through. When she got into his room, she saw that Jimmy had barricaded himself inside. He was hiding under piles of clothes and sheets, screaming about the government spy agencies. He said that the CIA was putting some thoughts into his head and taking other thoughts out. Jimmy said that every time a plane flew over the neighborhood, it meant that the CIA was manipulating his thoughts. Jimmy was petrified and inconsolable. His mother called 911, and, within minutes, police and emergency medical services were at the house.

When Jimmy arrived at the local hospital, he was still upset. He told the nurses and doctors everything he told his mother. The doctor offered Jimmy medications, but he refused and told the doctors that they might be working for the CIA. He started yelling in the emergency room and attracted significant attention. He was held down by hospital staff and administered haloperidol, an antipsychotic, 5 mg, and lorazepam, an antianxiety medication, 2 mg, intramuscularly. Jimmy settled down and then fell asleep for six hours. When he woke up, he was much calmer but continued to tell the doctors about his concerns about being monitored.

He was admitted to the psychiatric unit of the local hospital and diagnosed with "Psychotic Disorder, Not Otherwise Specified." Jimmy was initially prescribed risperidone, another antipsychotic, 1 mg twice daily. After two days, he continued to be calm and did not show any side effects to the medications. He was cooperative with his doctors but continued to talk about the CIA and NSA. He was also seen talking to himself in the common room of the unit. The doctors increased the risperidone to 2 mg twice a day. Jimmy's mother visited him every day, and, while she was concerned about his health, she was relieved to see he was getting better and finally received medical attention. Jimmy stopped speaking to himself and told the doctors that he had been hearing voices saying disturbing things like, "We know what you're going to do" and "We know who you are," but they went away. However, he still had vague feelings about being watched. The doctors increased the risperidone to 3 mg twice daily. Jimmy started to feel tired during the day.

After another week on the psychiatric unit, Jimmy told his mother and the doctors that he felt much safer. He no longer heard voices and did not believe the CIA was monitoring his thoughts. Jimmy had a meeting with the doctors and his mother. They told him that he suffered from schizophrenia, which, they explained, was a chronic illness without a cure. However, they explained that treatments did exist, including the medication he was currently taking and psychotherapy. When the doctors asked if anyone in Jimmy's family suffered from a mental illness, Jimmy's mother recalled that his father also acted unusually before he left the family, which happened when he was about Jimmy's age.

Jimmy was discharged from the hospital and given a follow-up appointment to see a psychiatrist in a clinic nearby. The psychiatrist decided to continue prescribing risperidone 3 mg twice daily, since Jimmy responded well to it, and he didn't have any serious side effects, except for feeling tired during the day, which the doctor said was normal.

Jimmy continued to live with his mother. He continued to see the outpatient psychiatrist and take his medication. Jimmy gained about 25 pounds which upset him and his mother, but they both agreed it was better than getting sick and going back to the hospital. After a year, Jimmy decided that he wanted to continue his studies and become an engineer. His psychiatrist encouraged him to follow his dreams but recommended that he start with one class at a time. Jimmy reenrolled at State and took a calculus course that is required for engineers.

After several weeks, Jimmy became extremely frustrated. He wasn't as good at math as he was in high school, and he started having thoughts that everyone else in the class knew he had schizophrenia. He thought the risperidone was making him duller and too tired to study as hard as he needed to. He stopped taking the medication and very quickly stopped sleeping. His mother noticed him speaking to himself and called his outpatient psychiatrist, who insisted that Jimmy come in for an urgent visit.

Jimmy's mother made sure that he started taking the medication again, and they both went to the appointment. Jimmy spoke about the stress of class and feeling like he isn't smart enough anymore. He was praised for his ambition and assured that his difficulty was due to a mental illness, not a lack of intelligence. He dropped his calculus course and spent the next several months sitting around the house, watching TV. His psychiatrist explained the importance of getting out of the house and using his time productively, but Jimmy felt dejected and couldn't think of anything he wanted to do.

Jimmy's mother thought hard about meaningful ways he could use his time. After looking and asking around, she found a neighborhood organization for people with schizophrenia and other major mental illnesses. The organization offered a wide variety of classes and activities for patients and their parents. Jimmy took several classes and then, with encouragement from his mother, took a leadership role in the organization. His role was to organize the kitchen that provided free meals to the clients. He often planned meals and helped cook them. His mother frequently cooked with him in the organization's kitchen. On special occasions, Jimmy and his mother made the same pastries for the clients that they made when Jimmy was growing up, which were *extremely* popular with the clients and organization staff.

Analysis

This vignette represents a typical onset and presentation of schizophrenia, a common psychotic disorder. Under the *Diagnostic and Statistical Manual,* Fifth Edition, which classifies mental illnesses and was published in 2013, there are no subtypes of schizophrenia, but Jimmy would have been diagnosed with schizophrenia, paranoid type (aka paranoid schizophrenia), under formal guidelines.

Most major mental illnesses, including schizophrenia, emerge in late adolescence and young adulthood. Jimmy shows signs of having a mental illness during his first semester of college, which is not uncommon. Patients have a variety of experiences prior to the full emergence of mental illness. Some have completely normal childhoods, without any sign that they may develop mental illness later in life. Some patients, like Jimmy, have difficulty fitting in or have interests that are generally not aligned with their peers.

Jimmy's initial symptoms of mental illness were typical of a prodromal syndrome. Before the onset of schizophrenia, patients generally go through a period of social withdrawal, anxiety, depression, and poor hygiene. This is an extremely difficult period for patients, as they have some sense that something is off in how they are thinking and feeling but do not know what it is and do not know what to do. It is very common for patients experiencing prodromal symptoms to experiment with substances, especially marijuana, as Jimmy did, to feel better or at least differently.

After Jimmy was home for several months, classic symptoms of schizophrenia fully emerged. He became delusional about government agencies, which are common subjects of paranoid thoughts. He also described thought insertion and thought deletion, which are the belief that thoughts are being put in and taken out of one's mind, respectively. In the hospital, Jimmy explained to the doctors that he experienced auditory hallucinations, which is a hallmark feature of schizophrenia.

When Jimmy was first in the emergency room, he was given haloperidol, an antipsychotic, and lorazepam, an antianxiety medication, intramuscularly. Staff held him down to give him the shot against his will. Administration of any medication against the patient's will is an extremely serious action, because it violates a patient's rights over his or her own body. However, it is legal, and medically and ethically justified, under certain circumstances. In this example, Jimmy was acutely paranoid and believed that doctors were involved with the spy agencies that were persecuting him. Although Jimmy was never a violent person by temperament, he may have seriously hurt hospital staff under the false belief that he was acting in self-defense. Therefore, it was necessary to sedate Jimmy to protect him and hospital staff.

After he received medications, he was calmer and willing to work with the doctors. He accepted medications by mouth, so injections were not necessary. While all patients have different responses to antipsychotics, Jimmy's quick recovery to risperidone, another antipsychotic, was not uncommon. Antipsychotics are generally very effective at decreasing the intensity of delusions and auditory hallucinations. They are less effective in addressing other symptoms of schizophrenia, including isolation, disorganized behavior, and poor hygiene.

It is very common for patients to stop taking antipsychotic medications. There are many reasons for this, including a denial of having a mental illness in the first place and the many difficult side effects of the medication. For example, the risperidone was making Jimmy tired and caused him to gain weight. Many hospitalizations of patients with schizophrenia are due to non-compliance with antipsychotic medications.

Ultimately, a schizophrenic patient's quality of life will be determined by the strength of his or her support network and how he or she spends his or her time. Unfortunately, many patients with schizophrenia do not have supportive families. This is partially due to the difficult nature of taking care of a loved one with a major mental illness. Also, as many mental illnesses, including schizophrenia, are hereditary, many patients' parents are also ill and unable to care for them (like Jimmy's father). Too often, patients with schizophrenia do not spend their time constructively because the lack of motivation and organization is a symptom of the illness. They are at risk of becoming dejected, hopeless, and depressed. For these reasons, substance abuse is extremely high in patients with schizophrenia.

There are many community advocacy groups, including National Alliance on Mental Illness (NAMI), which are extremely instrumental in preventing hopelessness and isolation in patients with serious mental illnesses. By becoming involved in this type of program, Jimmy will be productive with his time, have a strong sense of purpose, and a high quality of life.

CASE 2: BOBBY

Bobby has always required more of his mother's attention than his older brother. Now he is eight years old, and his mother is beyond overwhelmed. Everyone who knows him, including his mother and the teachers who complain about his behavior so much, all say that he is a good kid at heart. The problems start when Bobby doesn't get his way or when he's in a bad mood. When Bobby gets angry or frustrated, he is extremely difficult to help, and his temper tantrums are becoming more frequent and intense.

Bobby and his older brother, Stan, 16, have always lived with their mother. Their father is currently incarcerated and is unlikely to rejoin the family any-time soon. Bobby's brother was diagnosed with attention-deficit/hyperactivity disorder (ADHD) and has been treated successfully with stimulants by a psychiatrist in a local mental health clinic. Bobby's mother suffers from depression and anxiety and has been intermittently treated in therapy for years. Bobby's father has never been formally evaluated by a mental health professional, but he has a history of substance abuse and impulsive, dangerous behaviors, including the criminal activity that resulted in his present prison sentence.

Stan was diagnosed with ADHD when he was 13 years old. His difficulties started in sixth grade. Stan was always a good student, but he became unable to sit still. He left his seat in class frequently and disrupted the class. He was sent to the principal on a weekly basis, which was unusual for him. The school responded by giving Stan detention regularly. His mother noticed that Stan's behavior at home was different. He couldn't focus on one task and would talk through television shows, leave meals early, and couldn't follow directions. She brought him to the local clinic, and a psychologist diagnosed him with ADHD. An appointment with a psychiatrist was arranged, and she prescribed Ritalin, a common stimulant used to treat ADHD. Stan's mother and teachers were thrilled with his progress. His grades improved, and he stopped getting detention. He takes his medication every day but sometimes skips it when he's on vacation and doesn't have to focus so rigidly.

When Bobby started showing similar behavior at age five, his mother wasn't overly concerned. She thought it was odd that Bobby was so much younger than Stan when he first had difficulty with attention and behavior, but she was optimistic that he would improve, just as Stan did with medications. His mother brought Bobby into the same mental health clinic, and he was soon diagnosed with ADHD and started on Ritalin, at a lower dose, because he was younger and smaller than Stan. Bobby's behavior improved slightly, but his teachers still complained. Bobby would often leave his seat and bother his peers. He never followed directions at home or school. His dose of Ritalin was increased which helped his attention a little bit more. However, he was still disruptive in school. The thing that set Bobby off the most was being disciplined by authority figures. He hated when his mother yelled at him, but she was used to his reactions and knew how to speak to him to avoid conflicts. However, when adults at school, or camp, or any after-school activities were stern with Bobby, the situation would escalate into a nightmare.

Bobby started acting in ways Stan never did. When he didn't get his way or was told to do something he didn't want to do, he would scream as loud as he could, occasionally breaking down in tears. This was more common at school, but his mother noticed it too. Babysitters refused to return because Bobby would melt down when told it was bedtime. Bobby's mother spoke with his therapist, and she recommended instituting a strict policy of carrots and sticks. He would get presents when he would cooperate, and privileges would be removed when he had one of his temper tantrums, which were now infamous at his school and all around the neighborhood. These policies were ineffective, and his mother lost patience. She started doing what everyone cautioned against; she started giving into his demands to avoid problems.

Over the next year, his psychiatrist tried many different combinations of ADHD medications. He was taking large amounts of Adderall and a different medication called guanfacine. Those medications helped, but his teachers still complained about his behaviors. By the time he turned seven, his tantrums took on a dangerous quality. If he got really mad, he would hit, bite, and throw things. These behaviors baffled his teachers and his mother. When he was in a good mood, he was a very sweet little boy. His mother and his teachers walked on eggshells to avoid his outbursts. However, at a certain point, Bobby's playtime had to end, he had to go to bed, or he had to brush his teeth, which could precipitate fireworks.

Bobby's second grade teacher had no patience for his temper tantrums, neither did the new principal. Also, as Bobby got bigger, his bites and punches became more painful. During the first week of school, his teacher told him very sternly to sit down in his seat in a manner that he found bossy and mean. He refused, and when she approached him, he threw a pencil and a chair at her. The teacher called a security guard who brought Bobby to the principal's office. Bobby continued to kick and scream, and the principal called the ambulance, which brought Bobby to the local emergency room (ER). Bobby's mother was shocked when she found out and left work early to meet him at the hospital. She knew that he could get out of control, but she thought an ambulance was over the top. This was a disciplinary issue. Aren't hospitals supposed to be for medical emergencies? In the ER, Bobby was tearful and apologetic. He calmed down, and Bobby's mother took him home. They set up an extra session with Bobby's therapist, and Bobby was able to write down things he could have done differently.

Things were better at school for the couple weeks. Bobby continued to take his ADHD medications, which worked, but not nearly as well as they did for Stan. He still struggled with attention and found it difficult to follow complicated directions. When assigned a chore by his mother, she often found that he abandoned the task shortly after starting and found something else to do. Three weeks after he was taken to the ER, an argument in recess over the rules of a game set Bobby off again. He bit another student and was again taken to the principal's office. When the principal tried to talk to Bobby, he screamed about how he knew the rules and the other boy was wrong. He could not calm down, so the principal called the ambulance again, and his mother left work early, again. This time, she was angrier. The family was completely dependent on her salary, and she could not afford to lose her job.

Bobby's behavior continued. By the middle of the school year, she was leaving work early several times a month. Her boss was understanding, but she missed out on a promotion as a result. Bobby's mother started getting very embarrassed, especially by the time she knew all the doctors and nurses at the local ER by name. Even though they were nice to her, she felt like they saw her as an incompetent mother. Sometimes Bobby's mother would wait until the end of the work day to pick Bobby up at the ER, because she didn't want to miss too much work. Bobby would then sit in the ER for an entire day, which not only made him mad but sad as well. He started crying at home whenever his behavior was discussed. His mother understood that he was still the same good-natured boy, but he had no tolerance for frustration. When he became upset, he lost control over his actions, and the consequences were significantly impacting his academics, his time at home, his mother's career, and now, even his happiness.

During ongoing discussions about his behavior problems, his psychiatrist raised the idea of starting a medication called risperidone, an antipsychotic. The idea seemed outlandish to Bobby's mother. He wasn't "crazy," so why would he take an antipsychotic? The psychiatrist explained that antipsychotics help regulate mood and control behavioral outbursts. She said that the dose would be much lower than the doses used to treat adults with serious mental illnesses, like schizophrenia. Ultimately, the psychiatrist said, the decision would be Bobby's mother's. She thought about the devastating effects of his tantrums and was extremely tempted by the possibility that the medication could bring some relief. But the psychiatrist was candid about the side effects of that medication, including weight gain, sedation, dry mouth, breast budding in males, and even diabetes. How could she expose her son to those conditions? But how could she allow him to ruin his education and possibly jeopardize her job, on which the family was dependent for groceries and rent? Bobby's mother wrestled with the decision. She asked all of her friends and family for guidance and lost sleep over it.

About a month later, a particularly ugly temper tantrum at the supermarket motivated Bobby's mother to try the medication. Bobby's mother refused to buy a sugary breakfast cereal, and as a show of protest, Bobby lay down in the aisle, screamed, and flailed his arms and legs until he got his way. When his strategy proved unsuccessful, he knocked an entire row of cereal off the shelves onto the ground. By this time a crowd had gathered, and store workers asked Bobby's mother to leave and not come back.

Bobby's psychiatrist prescribed risperidone 0.5 mg at bedtime to start, in addition to his ADHD medications. He tolerated this well, but his mother found it a little harder to wake Bobby up in the morning. While Bobby's behavior was still problematic, he showed improvement. He was sent to the principal's office less, and his tantrums were less intense. They now usually stopped at yelling and rarely progressed to the biting and throwing things that alarmed the school previously. He still had a monthly meltdown with dangerous behaviors that prompted ambulance rides. His psychiatrist added 0.5 mg in the morning as well.

After a few weeks, Bobby's mother and teachers saw a significant change, but it wasn't all good. While his temper tantrums became rare, he also stopped interacting normally. He never raised his hand in class. He also stopped playing sports at recess and just wanted to side on the stairs and hang out by himself. He didn't seem sad exactly, but he did seem detached and subdued. At home it was the same story. He didn't speak with his mother or brother as much and just wanted to be left alone to watch TV. His appetite increased, which didn't bother his mother because she always thought he was a little too skinny.

His psychiatrist decided to move all the medication to bedtime. Instead of 0.5 mg in the morning and at bedtime, he started to take 1 mg at night. This change generally improved his daytime demeanor, but his mother had an awful time getting him out of bed. He was frequently late for school. However, once he did get to school, he interacted well with friends, participating in class, and playing his favorite recess games.

His appetite continued to be unusually large. He ate a normal dinner with the family at 5:30 but then wanted to eat another full meal before bed at nine o'clock. He gained 25 lbs. in three months. Now Bobby felt bad about himself and found that he was no longer one of the fastest boys in his class. The distribution of the weight was also strange. His belly got bigger, but he also gained weight in his chest. Other kids teased him for looking like a girl, and someone tagged him in a Facebook picture as "Booby Bobby," which absolutely mortified him.

He started fighting with his mother about the medication and sometimes pretended to swallow the pill and spit it out after his mother turned around. His mother knew when he didn't take his medication because she got a call from the school about bad behavior. Taking medications turned into a nightly argument that his mother dreaded, and she had second thoughts about her decision. Ultimately, she believed she had made the right choice, because she no longer had to leave work early, and Bobby was doing much better academically, since he was now able to consistently remain in class. However, she knew that her choice carried a price, and she hoped that over time, the medications would lead to a happier and more successful outcome for Bobby and the whole family.

Analysis

Bobby's scenario raises many of the questions that have been most difficult for child psychiatrists to answer. The idea of medicating children always bears an increased level of concern and scrutiny. Bobby's case involves the medication of two children. Stan was medicated for a relatively classic presentation of ADHD with stimulants, the long-accepted treatment of choice. His brother Bobby, however, was treated for symptoms of ADHD with the same class of medications but was also given antipsychotics to address his behavior problems.

Medicating children is controversial for several reasons. First, children's brains are still developing, and it is difficult to understand the effect that psychoactive medications will have. Furthermore, behaviors, personalities, temperaments, and attitudes change dramatically during childhood and adolescence until we reach adulthood. Many successful and well-adjusted adults consistently behaved inappropriately during childhood, and everyone behaved badly at some point. Bad behavior and dealing with consequences are the processes by which people learn social norms and etiquettes. There is concern that the medical community and society in general are "medicalizing" normal development and prescribing drugs, whose full effects we do not really understand, when children should be left alone to learn and grow without medications.

When stimulants became commonplace in the early 2000s, many people adopted similar attitudes and believed that ADHD was widely overdiagnosed and the stimulants overprescribed. Gradually, people have come to understand that ADHD can be very difficult for children and adolescents, and medical intervention is appropriate. Untreated ADHD can result in poor academic performance, which can lead to a decreased quality of life. Furthermore, ADHD can lead to poor self-esteem, depression, and substance abuse. As more people become aware of these facts, treatment for ADHD has become less controversial. According to the DSM-V, 5% of children suffer from ADHD.

However, Bobby's case was different. While he met criteria for ADHD, he also showed atypical behavior and symptoms. Psychiatrists have struggled to define behavior like that of Bobby and assign it to a specific diagnosis. When adults behave badly in the absence of another clear psychiatric problem, they are usually diagnosed with a personality disorder. However, personalities are not thought to be fully formed until 17 or 18 years of age, so it is generally not good practice to diagnose children with personality disorders. Many children like Bobby are diagnosed with opposition defiant disorder, which essentially describes problems with authority figures. It involves anger, irritability, argumentative behavior, and vindictiveness. However, the violent nature of Bobby's tantrums and the rapid mood swings go beyond this diagnosis. Children like Bobby are often diagnosed with intermittent explosive disorder, which is as the name implies. In many settings, Bobby may be diagnosed with bipolar disorder, mostly because of his dramatic mood swings. The idea behind giving children this diagnosis is that Bobby's volatile mood implies that he is likely to develop classic bipolar disorder, with episodes of depression and mania, later in life. Therefore, it would be helpful to make this diagnosis early and prescribe the appropriate medications as soon as possible. However, the result of this practice is likely an overdiagnosis of bipolar disorder in children with bad behavior. Once children have the diagnosis of bipolar disorder, they may be prescribed unnecessary medication well into adulthood before clinicians realize that bipolar disorder never developed. To address this problem, a diagnosis called disruptive mood dysregulation disorder was added to the DSM during the most recent edition (DSM-V 2013). It captures temper outbursts as a manifestation of a persistently irritable or angry mood and does not imply a lifelong mental illness like bipolar disorder. Bobby would not be included in this diagnosis, because when he is not having a temper tantrum and when he is not challenged by an authority figure, he is a lovely child. Therefore, his diagnoses would better be recorded as ADHD, oppositional defiant disorder, and intermittent explosive disorder.

As complicated as categorizing the behavior is, treating it is even more problematic. Ideally, educating parents and teachers about behavior modification techniques is the best solution. However, this is easier said than done. Bobby's mother tried this and failed miserably. Therefore, many parents and clinicians turn to medications. Several classes of medication have been used to address problematic behavior in children and adolescents, including selective serotonin reuptake inhibitors (SSRIs), typically used for depression, mood stabilizers like lithium or valproic acid, typically used for bipolar disorder, or antipsychotics, typically used for psychotic disorders like schizophrenia. As mentioned earlier, the dosages used to treat behavioral outburst in children are much less than those used to treat adult schizophrenia. For example, risperidone, is typically dosed at between 4 and 8 mg daily for adults with psychotic disorders. Bobby took 1 mg daily, which is a standard dose for someone of his age and presentation. Risperidone has a Food and Drug Administration (FDA) indication to treat aggression in children associated with autism, a diagnosis Bobby does not carry. Therefore, psychiatrists who prescribe risperidone and other antipsychotics to patients like Bobby do so "off-label."

When considering the use of a medication, like an antipsychotic, to reduce the intensity of temper tantrums, a careful risk/benefit analysis is necessary. As discussed in depth elsewhere in this text, antipsychotics have serious adverse effects. Generally, the tipping point when parents will opt for an antipsychotic is when temper tantrums become dangerous. If the temper tantrums are only annoying or embarrassing, many parents will suffer through them and wait for the child to grow out of them while using parenting techniques to the best of their ability. However, if temper tantrums involve dangerous behaviors like that of Bobby, parents may decide that it could be more harmful to the child and others not to use all available medications. These decisions are not easy, as seen by Bobby's mother's loss of sleep.

Unfortunately, many schools often resort to using emergency medical services to address students' behavioral outbursts. Occasionally this intervention is warranted, if the behaviors represent a manifestation of a serious mental illness that warrants hospitalization. However, some school administrators have too low of a threshold to involve ambulances and hospitals when teachers and guidance counselors may be able to de-escalate a situation. This practice is partially based on legal liability. If a school refers a misbehaving child to the ER, they are not liable for his or her actions. However, if a school does not respond by sending a child to the hospital and the child then injures another student, the school may be held responsible for damages. The result, however, has been increasingly crowded pediatric ERs, increased medical costs, and a diversion of medical resources from patients who actually need help. A class-action lawsuit was filed in New York City in 2014 on behalf of children whose civil rights were allegedly violated by being unnecessarily referred to ERs.

CASE 3: GEORGE

George was born in London into a highly distinguished British family. His parents had high hopes for George and arranged for a world-class education. He had widely respected tutors for many subjects, including arts, sciences, and humanities.

His education came in handy when he took over the family business at age 22, after his grandfather passed away (George's father died when he was 13). George was good at his job and was well liked. He married a pretty girl just before his promotion. They had a supportive and happy marriage and raised 15 children.

When George was 26, he became quite ill. He had a bad cough, chest pain, fever, fatigue, and lost weight as well. He slept very poorly, usually about two hours a night. He became preoccupied with his death and worried about who would take over the family business. His mind was so consumed that making important decisions was very difficult.

However, George got better in a few months and he was back to his old self. His job was stressful and when he was about 50, some of the men who worked for him decided to break off and start their own enterprise, which was not good for the bottom line.

When George was 50, he fell ill again with a similar sickness. He had bad abdominal pain and fevers for two weeks. This time, George's behavior changed in a way that concerned his family. He became agitated, spoke faster than normal, and couldn't focus on one topic. He slept poorly. At times, he was physically aggressive with his family and became preoccupied with sexual fantasies. At one point he tried to engage in sexual relations with his wife and daughter in public. This was extremely unusual for George, and the family brought in the best mental health professionals to treat him. He had to take several months off from work to relax, and even when he felt better, his work schedule was markedly decreased.

He had a couple more bouts of this illness over the next several years, but none was as serious. When he was 70, he had an eye infection that got so bad he became blind.

Despite several other setbacks, the company grew and George was a well-respected boss. He was the leader longer than anyone who had previously ran the family business. When he was 72, George's youngest and favorite daughter died, which completely devastated him. During her illness, he stayed in her room and cried every day. His melancholy was so severe that it was difficult for friends and family to see.

After that, he became ill again and remained so for the last 10 years of his life. While there were some lucid and calm moments, for the most part, his behavior and thoughts were clearly disordered. George became unable to function in his capacity as the head of such a large organization, and he was forced to resign. His son, who was also named George, took over.

He spoke fast and often either incomprehensibly or about inappropriate topics. He slept for one or two hours per night, and it was speculated that he heard voices that other people did not hear. He gradually lost intellectual ability, and his communications with his family became more simple and unsophisticated. He died surrounded by his family.

George would have benefited from antipsychotics during his most extreme episodes, but he was born in 1738, over 200 years before their development.

Analysis

The astute reader may have identified George as King George III of England (1738–1820). George is most commonly known, at least in the United States, for having ruled England during the American Revolution. He is also famous for having suffered the illness described previously, whose descriptions are quoted from the many nurses and physicians who cared for George. His psychiatric symptoms were made famous by the movie and play *The Madness of King George*.

There is much debate about the exact diagnosis or diagnoses that plagued George. Of course, it is impossible to make a definitive medical conclusion without a complete medical and psychiatric examination. However, while George had severe symptoms of mental illness at various points in his life, including depression, anxiety, psychosis, and dementia, his illness was most likely not primarily psychiatric. Applying modern medical standards to documentation of George's experience, it is widely believed that he suffered from acute intermittent porphyria (AIP) or a closely related condition. AIP is a metabolic disorder affecting the synthesis of heme, which is the central component of hemoglobin, which is largely responsible for oxygenating blood. Common symptoms include abdominal pain, urinary symptoms, numbness, tingling, weakness, and, of course, several psychiatric symptoms. Others believe that George's psychiatric condition had little or nothing to do with any physical problems and that he suffered from late-onset bipolar disorder.

This clinical vignette was included to demonstrate an error that was common in George's time but also persists today. George was considered "mad" by many, because the connection between mind and body was not well understood. There are many medical illnesses that are not directly related to the brain or even central nervous system, in which psychiatric problems can be some of the most prominent symptoms. Examples include thyroid disease, infection, and cancer. Therefore, it is absolutely critical that physicians, including ER doctors, primary care doctors, and psychiatrists, consider a wide possibility of diagnoses, even if a patient describes symptoms that are consistent with a primary psychiatric disorder, like schizophrenia or major depressive disorder. If a physician were to assume that everyone with hallucinations had schizophrenia, he or she would misdiagnose people like George. AIP is treatable with several medications and nutritional supplements.

However, there is still a role for antipsychotics in the treatment of patients with psychiatric symptoms of diseases that are not primarily related to mental health. In George's case, antipsychotics would most likely have been useful in decreasing George's hallucinations and paranoia. They also would have made him less anxious and help him eat and sleep better. Nonetheless, as his problem was not primarily psychiatric, the AIP would remain untreated. George would still suffer from abdominal pain, weakness, urinary symptoms, and any psychiatric problems that are not treated by antipsychotics. Therefore, the optimal way to address patients with psychiatric symptoms whose root cause is unclear is to treat the illness with psychiatric medications but continue to investigate the true nature of the illness.

There are several clues that mental health problems may be caused by medical problems unrelated to the mind. The first thing to consider is any feature of the patient's presentation that is not consistent with a typical presentation of the associated mental illness. For example, auditory hallucinations and paranoia are common symptoms of schizophrenia, which generally develops in young adults between 18 and 25 years old. Therefore, if a 60-year-old male complains about voices and thoughts that his wife is poisoning him, the responsible physician will have a strong suspicion that there may be a medical problem, like a brain tumor. Also, if the psychiatric symptoms occur simultaneously to other somatic problems, it is possible that all the symptoms are part of one medical illness. If a patient goes to an ER and his family explains that he began experiencing hallucinations in the same week as severe abdominal pain, weakness, and pain during urination, a reasonable doctor would consider AIP instead of directly automatically diagnosing a primary psychotic disorder, like schizophrenia. No matter how that doctor wishes to proceed in the diagnostic process, antipsychotics should be given to relieve upsetting psychiatric symptoms in the short term. Despite widely available knowledge of medical illnesses that are associated with mental health manifestations, many such patients are misdiagnosed with mental illnesses and their true disease remains untreated.

Chapter 2

What Are Antipsychotics?

Antipsychotics are a class of psychiatric medication traditionally used to treat psychosis, more specifically, the debilitating symptoms that are a product of the altered state. They were introduced in the United States in the 1950s and have gone through many changes and developments in both use and production since that time. They are sometimes referred to as psychotropics or neuroleptics. The term "neuroleptic" comes from the Greek *lepsis*, meaning to seize or take hold. As will be discussed in further detail later on, antipsychotics are used primarily to treat psychosis, and the term "neuroleptic" is a description of the drug "seizing" or "taking hold of" the patient's cognition and behavior and attempting to return the patient to a more reality-based state. Similarly, a psychotropic refers to anything that acts on and alters the mind. The term "psychotropic" is a more general and inclusive term to describe many, if not all, of the medications that are used to treat various psychiatric disorders. This chapter will serve to explore what antipsychotics are through a generalized lens, and many of the following chapters will then delve into various aspects of antipsychotics in greater detail. However, in order to have an understanding of what these medications are, one must first have a grasp on why they were needed, what drove their development, and the types of illnesses or symptoms they were and are still aimed at treating.

PSYCHOTIC DISORDERS AND THE SYMPTOMS OF PSYCHOSIS

Psychosis is a broad term that describes an alteration of one's state of reality. The term "psychotic" can be used to describe a manifestation of a psychiatric illness, but there are many other causes of psychosis, including, but not limited to, prescription drug induced, illicit substance induced, and induced by a general medical condition. The term "psychotic" is broad, and similarly the symptoms that "psychotic" describes are wide-ranging. It does not paint a clear picture to simply say that a person is psychotic. There must be a more detailed description and explanation of the person's symptoms in order to get an accurate understanding of what the nature of the psychosis is. Although the symptoms are wide-ranging, there are some classic symptoms that are associated with certain psychiatric illnesses. The next few paragraphs will be devoted to a brief discussion of some of the more commonly seen psychotic symptoms. Included will be clinical vignettes to demonstrate those symptoms as a manifestation in some of the classic psychiatric psychotic disorders. In a later chapter of the book, there will be a more detailed review of specific psychiatric disorders that are treated with antipsychotics and how they are diagnosed according to the *Diagnostic and Statistical Manual of Mental Disorders*.

The symptoms of psychosis can initially be broken into two large categories: positive symptoms and negative symptoms. Positive symptoms describe an individual's way of speaking, way of thinking, and any disturbances in perception. They are the symptoms that are generally most noticeable to the public and most behaviorally disturbing. They can be thought of as symptoms (thought processes and feelings) that are added on to the individual's baseline. The positive symptoms will be discussed in more detail later. The negative symptoms of psychosis pertain to an individual's affect, which is how the individual shows emotion, and cognition. These symptoms cause a slowing, with decreased motivation, and can be thought of as a taking away from an individual's baseline. The negative symptoms will be discussed in further detail when examining the specific effects that antipsychotics have in various disorders. The positive symptoms of psychosis can be broken up into three broad categories: delusions, perceptual disturbances, and thought disorders.

Delusions

A delusion is a fixed, false belief that cannot be changed even when confronted by reason or actual fact. The delusion cannot be accounted for by the cultural background of the individual. Delusions can be thought of as falling into four general categories and then can be further subtyped. Initially they can be thought of as bizarre, non-bizarre, mood-congruent, or mood neutral. Delusions often manifest themselves in consistent themes and can be understood in thematic categorization. Some common examples of delusions include:

- Delusions of persecution/paranoid delusions: "The other students at school are poisoning my food, so I haven't eaten at school in 1 week." "The CIA has been following me for years and has implanted a chip in my body in order to control me."
- Delusions of control: Includes thought broadcasting, which is the belief that one's thoughts can be heard by others. "I am not going to answer that question. I know you already know what I am thinking. Everybody knows what I am thinking." It also includes thought insertion, which is the belief that others place their thoughts in the individual's head. "I wasn't thinking about harming that person on the street, but my mother keeps putting these thoughts in my head."
- Delusions of grandeur: "I am the Son of God and have come to lead you to eternal greatness. I am all-powerful on earth and rewarded on earth and beyond with great powers and many wives."
- Ideas of reference: Belief that events or remarks in everyday environment have special meaning to that individual. "Well today when I was reading the newspaper I read a story that I am sure was written about me."
- Delusions of guilt: "It is because of me that so many people have died in that horrible hurricane."
- Delusion of jealousy: "I know that he has been seeing someone else. I can just tell because he has been checking his phone more often at home and saying hello to me in a different way."
- Somatic delusions: "I know that I am dying because I have become infested with worms that are devouring my internal organs."

The following "clinical vignette" exemplifies paranoid/persecutory delusions. The patient is paranoid that the Central Intelligence Agency (CIA) and his mother are constantly watching him and possibly trying to harm him. It also touches on delusions of grandeur as the patient has a delusion about how powerful he is and how this affects his relationship with the CIA.

Mr. S is a 35-year-old male who has been seeing an outpatient psychiatrist for the past seven years. He has been psychiatrically hospitalized three times in the past seven years, and tonight he has been brought into the emergency department by his mother whom he lives with. His mother states lately he has been saying "odd things at home and just isn't making very much sense."

Dr.: Mr. S. how have things been at home lately?

Mr. S: Things are not good. I don't understand why they are always watching me. Always watching.

Dr.: That sounds frightening. Who is always watching?

Mr. S: The CIA. They are everywhere, know everything I do. They even have cameras in the house. And I think they have gotten to my mom.

Dr.: What makes you say that?

Mr. S: I can just tell by the way she is looking at me. She is in on it with them. And now she is trying to poison my food.

Dr.: Do you think there is a reason that the CIA is interested in watching you?

Mr. S: Yes

Dr.: Why is that?

Mr. S: They know that I have the answers to the unbreakable codes. That I am the most powerful man on Earth.

Perceptual Disturbances

A perceptual disturbance is a sensory disturbance in the way one perceives his or her own surroundings. These disturbances can be classified into two main categories: illusions and hallucinations. Illusions are a misinterpretation of real external stimuli. It is a sensory distortion and therefore can occur with most senses but is most commonly visual, auditory, or tactile. For example, an individual sees a shadow and mistakes it for a person (visual). In another example, a person has had an amputation of the right arm but has the sensation that the arm still exists. This refers to a phantom limb, which is a tactile illusion.

Hallucinations are sensory perceptions without external stimuli. Again these can occur with various senses; however, auditory hallucinations are most common in the classic psychiatric psychotic disorders such as schizophrenia, bipolar disorder, and major depressive disorder.

- Auditory hallucination: "I hear a man's voice telling me to walk into moving traffic." Commonly seen in schizophrenia and other psychotic mental illnesses.
- Visual hallucination: "I was seeing spiders crawling all over the walls." These are less common in schizophrenia or bipolar disorder. Visual hallucinations are more commonly seen in intoxication, withdrawal states, and some general medical conditions (delirium and some dementias).
- Olfactory hallucination: "I smell something burning, but no one around me does." This commonly occurs as an aura associated with epilepsy.

- Tactile hallucination: "I feel like there are little bugs crawling up and down my arms!" Seen most often in drug abuse and alcohol withdrawal.

The following "clinical vignette" exemplifies auditory hallucinations, one of the perceptual disturbances. In this example, the patient expresses hearing two voices that are persecutory in nature. The doctor should ask more follow-up questions about the voices, like how often she hears them, if she recognizes the voices, and if there is anything she can do to make them go away. Not all auditory hallucinations are distressing to patients, and some patients are happy to go on living with them. There are actually networks (one of which is the Hearing Voices Network) that embrace their hallucinations and do not treat them as a chronic illness. Instead, they develop alternative approaches to coping with emotional distress.

Ms. B is a 40-year-old female who has struggled with depression since she was in her mid-20s. For the past three weeks she has been severely depressed, not wanting to get out of bed or enjoy her normal activities. She has been fired from her job and lost 15 lbs. She brought herself into the emergency department because she was having thoughts of suicide.

Dr.: Ms. B, when was the last time you had a thought about hurting yourself?

Ms. B: The last time I thought it on my own was a few days ago.

Dr.: What do you mean, the last time you thought it on your own? Is someone else suggesting you harm yourself?

Ms. B: These 2 voices I keep hearing. One is a female voice that tells me I am worthless and useless. The other is a male voice that comes up with ideas for how I should do it. He often tells me I should just go to the bridge and end it all.

Thought Disorders

Thought disorder refers to the form of speech as opposed to the content of the speech. It characterizes disorganized thinking that the patient does not show an awareness of. There are different types of formal thought disorder that can be seen is various psychotic disorders, most often schizophrenia and bipolar disorder. Provided next are some examples of thought disorders. It is important to keep in mind that some of the following examples can be seen during times of extreme stress and are not necessarily indicative of a disorder. However it is the severity, frequency, and resulting functional impairment that must be considered when observing speech patterns that are framed in a context of other symptoms.

- Circumstantiality: The person answers questions but adds extra and irrelevant details. "Where do you live?" "When I was a child I lived on the east coast and I liked it there, but eventually just decided that it wasn't really for me. So for a little while when I was in my 20s I tried out the west coast. It was a good time for me to be out there. I really enjoyed the ocean and just the lifestyle and the mind-set of people out there. I stayed there for a while. Eventually though I had to move because of my job and now I live in Oklahoma."
- Tangentiality: The person does not answer the question directly and never comes to the point of the conversation. The conversation is usually about similar material but lacks goal-directed associations. "Where do you live?" "When I was a child I lived on the east coast and I liked it there, but eventually just decided that it wasn't really for me. So then I moved out to the west coast when I was in my 20s. It was a good time for me to be out there. I really enjoyed the ocean and just the lifestyle and the mind-set of the people out there. I don't think some people can go from the east coast pace to the west coast pace but I really felt like it fit me well. I stayed there for a while and that's where I met my good friend Claudia."
- Flight of ideas: The individual switches from topic to topic rapidly and it is often accompanied by pressured speech that cannot be interrupted. This is often seen in the manic phase of bipolar disorder. "I have not been sleeping very much lately because I just have too much on my mind. When I have too much on my mind I just don't have time to do anything else. Sometimes I don't even eat. I like eating though. My favorite food is mashed potatoes. But sometimes I like ice cream more. Especially when the weather is hot. I really do like the summer time much more than the winter."
- Neologisms: A person inserts made-up words into otherwise normal sentences.
- Word salad: The speech is largely incoherent, however, it is spoken in regular rhythm and prosody usually.
- Thought blocking: An individual stops in mid-sentence and cannot continue his or her thought; the silence can last a few seconds to longer than a minute.

The next "clinical vignette" exemplifies a patient with flight of ideas in an acute manic state. He is jumping from topic to topic rapidly. He is also speaking fast, and the doctor is unable to interrupt his words or thoughts. It also touches again on delusions of grandeur, which are common in manic states. This patient thinks he is a famous rapper and will be a famous poet.

Mr. T is a 22-year-old male who has never seen a psychiatrist before. He was brought in by his father because for the past four days he has not been sleeping at all. He has been up throughout the night and has started many new projects at home but cannot seem to complete any of them. His father also says that he sounds different than normal, and he is having a hard time understanding what he is saying.

Dr.: Hi Mr. T, how are you doing today?

Mr. T: Hi doc, I am on top of the world, better than ever. A feeling I can't describe. I can describe a lot of things. Part of the reason why I am such a good writer. I think I am going to be a famous poet someday. Maybe a rapper too. Have you ever been a poet? In fact I already am a famous rapper. Maybe you have heard of me? T-timing? I wrote some lyrics here if you want to see them. Lyrics are funny right? Just the thoughts that come to my head but they are so good. I have a lot of thoughts. Different thoughts all the time. Time is a funny thing too.

Dr.: I see you have . . . (unable to interrupt)

Mr. T: Sometimes time goes very fast and other times so slow. I like it when it goes by fast. I like moving fast, you know? Like fast cars.

TREATMENT OF PSYCHOSIS: FROM EXORCISM TO ANTIPSYCHOTICS

Psychotic symptoms and disorders have been documented since early civilization. However, society's view of and approach to treatment have changed drastically over the centuries. In early civilizations, psychosis was thought to be caused by the supernatural. There is evidence from human skulls suggesting that in ancient times there was an attempt to cure psychosis by drilling a hole into the skull in order to release the spirits that had inhabited the brain. Other groups used exorcism, and some still do to this day, in order to rid the inflicted of the "demons" that were causing these symptoms. It was Hippocrates who proposed a natural cause of psychosis and viewed health through a holistic lens. He suggested that medicine must address ailments not only of the body but of the mind as well. This led to the practice of bloodletting as Hippocrates thought that diseases were caused by an imbalance in various bodily fluids. Psychotic symptoms were thought to be caused by an excess of blood, so the practice of bloodletting was used in attempt to improve psychosis. In the early 20th century, the focus of treatment shifted from addressing bodily fluids to shocking the nervous system, most notably through electroconvulsive therapy. The various forms of "shock therapy" at that time came with considerable risk but were noted to have great effects, particularly upon schizophrenia. The acceptance of these high-risk treatments led to exploration of even higher risk treatments such as psychosurgery. These surgeries encompassed various operations, including removal of the cerebral cortex and the well-known prefrontal lobotomy. While these surgeries were very high-risk and controversial, the lobotomy became widespread as there seemed to be no alternative until about the 1950s when antipsychotics were introduced.

Antipsychotics, of course, have their own history of development and transformation, which will be discussed in detail in the next chapter. Chlorpromazine was the first antipsychotic approved for the treatment of acute and chronic psychosis in the early 1950s; however, at that time its mechanism of action was unknown and would not be discovered for another decade. Between 1954 and 1975 more than 10 different antipsychotics were introduced in the United States and dozens were introduced worldwide. All of these antipsychotics were in the same class and had a similar side effect profile and are now referred to as the "typical" antipsychotics. There was then a long break in the United States with no introduction of new antipsychotics until 1989 when clozapine, the first "atypical" antipsychotic, was introduced in the United States.

The first antipsychotics are phenothiazine derivatives, which are organic tricyclic compounds soluble in acetic acid, benzene, and ether and found in the synthetic dye, methylene blue. Many antipsychotic and antihistamine medications are derivatives from the phenothiazine compound.

Chlorpromazine and its predecessors were first observed to be useful as anesthetics and were used for sedation during clinical procedures. Interestingly, it was observed that in patients taking chlorpromazine, as opposed to some of the other similar derivatives being used as anesthetics, there was no loss of consciousness, but instead it seemed to induce sleepiness and brought on apathy. Patients that were taking chlorpromazine showed a lack of interest in events that were occurring around them and to them. After these observations were made, it was thought that this medication may be useful to help subdue some of the psychiatric patients who showed hyperactive, agitated, or aggressive behaviors. So while it is likely that some of the first uses of chlorpromazine in psychiatry were for psychotic patients, the drug was initially used to target and control unwanted and undesirable behaviors in order to make patients more suitable for discharge from hospitals. Prior to the advent of antipsychotics, patients spent decades in state hospitals and would often live out their lives there. After the introduction of chlorpromazine, there was a large surge in discharges from state hospitals. With the medication, patients' behaviors became more socially acceptable, and they were deemed able to function in society. But still, the exact mechanism of action and understanding of the effects that the drug was having on the central nervous system would not come for years following.

After chlorpromazine was such a clinical success, there was a widespread search around the world for other antipsychotic medications. Over the next few decades, dozens of phenothiazine derivatives were developed that were similarly effective in treating psychosis but had slightly different chemistries, potencies, and side effect profiles. As these medications were introduced and their use became more popular, some of their less desirable side effects began to be seen and became somewhat understood. A large number of people who were taking these typical antipsychotic agents were noted to be experiencing a specific set of movement disorders called extrapyramidal symptoms. The number of patients who would develop these movements was so high that people began to think that these side effects were linked to the ability of the medications to be efficacious. It was thought that in order for antipsychotics to reach their full potential in reducing psychotic symptoms, the medication doses needed to be increased until extrapyramidal symptoms were seen. With time, people began to challenge this idea and began to try to develop a new set of medications. Researchers developed a new antipsychotic that was just as effective with little to no movement side effects. This medication was called clozapine, the first in a set of new antipsychotic drugs called atypical antipsychotics. While clozapine was thought to be associated with little to no extrapyramidal symptoms, it came with its own set of issues. First, while some researchers felt you could have an effective antipsychotic without extrapyramidal symptoms, others were still convinced that the two were linked and immediately dismissed clozapine. Second, there were reports from Finland that there was a life-threatening blood disorder called agranulocytosis that was associated with clozapine. It was introduced to the market and then quickly withdrawn because of these concerns. Some had already observed that it seemed to be extremely effective in a set of treatment-resistant patients, so more research was conducted on the medication, and it was eventually introduced to the U.S. market in 1990.

The antipsychotics thus far had been working well on the positive symptoms of schizophrenia such as hallucinations, delusions, and disorganized behavior and speech. However, they had not been known to have any effect on the other symptoms of schizophrenia, the negative symptoms. These symptoms include inactivity, poverty of thought and speech, flattening of affect, and social withdrawal. While the positive symptoms can be quite disruptive, if the negative symptoms are not addressed they can be extremely debilitating and often keep patients from being able to function independently in society. Therefore, there was a hope to develop antipsychotics that would not only address the positive symptoms but also help to diminish the negative symptoms. After clozapine was introduced, it was quickly noticed to have effect on both the positive and negative symptoms without the movement side effects. This discovery caused the belief that the effectiveness of antipsychotics was linked to movement side effects to be called into question. Soon there was a new concept about clozapine. It was thought to be the first of a new class of antipsychotics called "atypical antipsychotics" that worked on positive and negative symptoms and that did not often induce the extrapyramidal side effects. This led to the development of various other atypical antipsychotics in the 1990s. These medications became used as first-line choices over the typical antipsychotics, largely because of the side effect profiles. The development of new antipsychotics has continued to be based on the atypical antipsychotics.

However, as time has gone by and all of the antipsychotics have been used more and studied more, the distinction between the two classes has been somewhat blurred. While some still feel strongly that the atypical antipsychotics are superior to the typical antipsychotics in their efficacy and side effect profiles, others have suggested that atypical antipsychotics have a similar propensity to cause movement side effects. While these medications are largely divided into two classes, each has a slightly different profile that should be considered when trying to decide which medication to use in various circumstances. In order to have a greater understanding of antipsychotics as a whole, it is important to understand each of the medications individually.

TYPICAL ANTIPSYCHOTICS: THE BEGINNING

All typical antipsychotics work on dopamine receptors in various parts of the brain. One of the main current hypotheses about schizophrenia and other psychotic disorders is that they are caused by an excess of dopamine, at least in part of the brain. The typical antipsychotics work to treat psychotic symptoms by blocking those dopamine receptors and thus decreasing the amount of dopamine in the brain. Of course, it is slightly more complicated than that, but the mechanism of antipsychotics and how they work on the brain and have effects in various other parts of the body will be discussed in detail in a later chapter. As mentioned earlier, some of the typical antipsychotics are phenothiazine derivatives. The individual chemical makeup of these specific derivatives varies based on the side chain attached to the phenothiazine. But, not all of the typical antipsychotics are derived from the same chemical compound. There are a number of typical antipsychotics derived from various other chemical compounds such as butyrophenones, thioxanthenes, and dihydroindolones.

All of the typical antipsychotics, however, work as dopamine blockers, and they are classified not by the receptors they work on or their chemical structure but based on their potency. The potency of a medication refers to how much of the medication is needed in order to produce a specific effect. For instance, if you need 5 mg of drug x to cause a resolution of symptoms and 10 mg of drug y to cause the same resolution, then drug x is twice as potent as drug y. The typical antipsychotics are grouped into low potency, mid potency, and high potency, and in the following pages, each group will be looked at in closer detail. There are dozens of typical antipsychotics that have been developed and used in various parts of the country and the world, some more than others. In order to get a more complete understanding of this group of medications, it is important to have an understanding of some individual medications in the various potency groups and how to potentially apply them to a clinical setting.

Low Potency

All of the typical antipsychotics are thought to have relatively similar efficacy, meaning that at the optimized dose all of the typicals will be able to achieve similar results. The low potency antipsychotics have a weaker attraction to the dopamine receptors than the other antipsychotics. Therefore, in order to reach an effective dose when using the low potency medications, a higher dose will be required. While the antipsychotics' primary goal is to reduce the amount of dopamine in the brain, they certainly have effects on other receptors as well. The effects on other receptors lead to different side effects, prominently, anticholinergic and antihistaminic. Since they need to reach high doses in order to achieve antipsychotic effectiveness, they also will have a strong side effect profile based on the other receptors that will be targeted with the high doses. Antihistamines are a class of medication that are readily accessible and can be picked up at the local over-the-counter pharmacy. They are often used to help relieve allergic reactions. Benadryl is an example of an antihistamine used to relieve allergies. Blocking histamine receptors also can cause people to become sleepy. So with higher doses of low potency antipsychotics and more antihistamine activity, people will experience more sedation. One could imagine that when a person is psychotic, there are times that using medications that cause sleepiness and slowness could be quite beneficial and therapeutic. These situations will be discussed in further detail later on. While it seems that a sedating side effect could be beneficial, there are unfortunately other properties that come along with antihistamine and anticholinergic action that are less desirable. Antihistamines have long been associated with weight gain, and it is seen that the low potency antipsychotics (with more antihistaminergic properties) cause more weight gain than the high potency (with less antihistaminergic properties). Similarly, the low potency antipsychotics also work on cholinergic receptors leading to greater anticholinergic effects. Anticholinergics block acetylcholine in the nervous system (both in the brain and in the periphery). They inhibit nerves that control involuntary movements in different parts of the body, including the gastrointestinal tract, the urinary tract, and lungs. These medications have a role in treating some medical conditions, but when these transmitters are blocked in a person who did not have a need to block them, they can cause some unwanted side effects. These effects are more prominent with low potency antipsychotics because the doses have to be higher to reach effective antipsychotic range. The unwanted anticholinergic effects range in their severity and include such things as dry mouth, constipation, blurry vision, increased heart rate, decreased blood pressure, and urinary retention.

One of the more positive qualities of the low potency typicals is that they have been thought to have a lower incidence of the movement side effects that were described earlier with some of the antipsychotics. It has been thought that the reason they have less of a tendency for the movement side effects is because they have a weaker attraction for the dopamine receptors in the brain. While dopamine blockade is helpful for some of the psychotic symptoms, dopamine plays a major role in regulating many of our movements. It is the blockade of dopamine in other pathways in the brain that leads to the movement side effects. Since the low potency medications have a lower affinity for the dopamine receptors that are responsible for the psychotic symptoms, they likely also have a lower affinity for the receptors causing the unwanted movement side effects. One of the most used and well-known typical antipsychotics is a low potency medication, chlorpromazine.

Chlorpromazine

As mentioned earlier, chlorpromazine was the first antipsychotic approved on the market. It was first used in the 1950s and can be cited as the cause of one of the greatest advances in psychiatric care, leading to huge decreases in inpatient psychiatric hospitalizations. Its generic name is chlorpromazine, and it often goes by the trade name of Thorazine in the United States. Like many of the other low potency typicals, chlorpromazine has a broad effect. Its primary use is for psychotic symptoms. However, it has a broad range of actions, which causes it to have many side effects. This can make it difficult to use at times. Its broad range of actions also leads it to be used for other purposes than its antipsychotic properties, some of which will be discussed in the following paragraphs.

Therapeutics. Chlorpromazine's antipsychotic properties come from its ability to block dopamine receptors. It usually will cause improvement in psychotic symptoms within one week, but full effect on behavioral changes may take longer. It does not usually eliminate psychotic symptoms in people with a long-term psychotic illness like schizophrenia, but it will reduce the symptoms.

Side Effects. Chlorpromazine can cause movement side effects by blocking the dopamine receptors in a part of the brain (striatum) that plays a role in regulating movement. It blocks acetylcholine receptors giving an anticholinergic effect that can cause sedation, blurred vision, constipation, and dry mouth. Chlorpromazine also works on histamine receptors. By blocking the histamine receptors, it can cause sedation and weight gain. It also works on adrenergic receptors, which are involved in regulating the nervous system. By blocking adrenergic receptors, it leads to a slowing down of the peripheral nervous system, which can cause decreases in blood pressure and dizziness.

Dosing and Usage. Chlorpromazine is available in pill form, liquid, injectable, and suppository. Low doses are sometimes used for short-term relief of agitation. The normal dosing range to relieve long-term psychotic symptoms is somewhere between 200 and 800 mg per day. The medication does not have any qualities that would make it habit forming or addictive, but the medication should not be stopped abruptly. Instead, it should be slowly decreased over about six to eight weeks before stopping. If chlorpromazine is stopped abruptly, it can cause a rebound psychosis. If this occurs, a person who may be doing quite well on the medication could have a reoccurrence of his or her psychotic symptoms. Often these symptoms come back stronger and are more debilitating than the original symptoms.

Advantages and Disadvantages. While chlorpromazine is in a class with other antipsychotics that act similarly, it does have some specific properties that make it more suitable in certain situations. Chlorpromazine comes in a formulation that can be given as an injectable. This can be helpful when a person is acutely agitated and unable or unwilling to take a pill. Chlorpromazine can be put into a syringe and injected into the muscle. As mentioned previously, it is also quite sedating; so similarly, in a situation where a person is acutely agitated and may be dangerous to themselves or other people, chlorpromazine can be helpful in calming them down to keep them safe. Some of its properties that cause it to be advantageous can also be disadvantages in certain situations and with certain populations. For instance, its sedating properties could be unwanted in certain age groups, like children or the elderly. Chlorpromazine is well known to cause decreases in blood pressure, more so than some of the other medications in its category. The elderly are already generally prone to falling, and giving them a medication that makes them sleepy and could decrease their blood pressure puts them at a high risk for falling and causing other injuries to themselves. As a group, the low potency antipsychotics are thought to cause more heart problems than the other antipsychotics. They can cause a prolongation of one of the intervals of the heart's electrical cycle; this is called QTc prolongation. If this interval is prolonged too much, it can cause the heart to stop.

FDA-Approved Uses.   Chlorpromazine has been approved by the Food and Drug Administration (FDA) for many different uses. It has been approved for multiple different psychotic disorders, including schizophrenia, psychosis in mania (as part of bipolar disorder), and general psychosis that could be secondary to any cause. It is also approved for some behavioral management, including combativeness and/or explosive hyperexcitable behavior in children and children who show excessive motor hyperactivity with symptoms of impulsivity, aggressivity, and poor frustration tolerance. As mentioned before, it is anticholinergic and this property makes it helpful in nausea and vomiting, which it has been approved to treat. It is also approved to treat intractable hiccups. After examining the varied list of FDA-approved uses for chlorpromazine, it becomes clear that it has a broad range of actions. If it were more specific and could target specific symptoms, it would not create so many various effects. However, it reaches many different neurotransmitter systems, which is why it has been found useful in treating many different ailments.

Off-Label Uses.   Like many of the other medications that are commonly used, chlorpromazine has multiple FDA-approved uses but has also been known to be used to treat disorders or symptoms that it is not approved for. When using a medication to treat a non-FDA-approved disease, it is called off-label use. One of chlorpromazine's off-label uses is for maintenance of bipolar disorder. It was mentioned earlier that the medication is approved for mania in bipolar disorder, but it is not approved for continued use once a person is no longer in a manic episode. It is also occasionally used off-label to treat severe migraines. In Germany, it is used to treat insomnia and severe itchiness and is used prior to anesthesia (how it was originally discovered).

Thioridazine

Thioridazine is another low potency typical antipsychotic that is used much less frequently than chlorpromazine. Thioridazine is the generic medication, which is still available in the United States but is not considered a first-line treatment for psychosis. Its brand name is Mellaril, which was actually discontinued worldwide in 2005 due to concerns about its toxic effect on the heart and the eye.

Therapeutics. Thioridazine's antipsychotic properties come from its ability to block dopamine in the brain. Similar to chlorpromazine, the psychotic symptoms should show some improvement within about a week, but it may take longer to show full behavioral effects. It is not considered first-line, meaning it should be tried only after other antipsychotics have been tried because of its risky side effect profile.

Side Effects. Like chlorpromazine, this medication takes action on acetylcholine and histamine casing similar side effects of sedation, weight gain, dry mouth, constipation, and blurry vision. It is unique in the severity of some of its more dangerous side effects, and it is known for its potential toxicity to the heart. It was mentioned earlier that chlorpromazine can prolong one of the intervals of electricity of the heart, the QT interval. This is a side effect that is possible with most of the antipsychotics but is more common and more severe in some. In thioridazine, there is a dose-dependent prolongation of that interval, meaning that as the dose of thioridazine gets higher, the patient is at a higher risk of prolonging the QT interval leading to cardiac arrest. Another side effect that is specific to thioridazine is the deposition of pigment in the retina of the eye leading to eventual blindness. This side effect also seems to be dose-dependent and is seen in patients taking doses over the recommended amount.

Dosing and Usage. Thioridazine is available in tablet and liquid form. It is generally thought best to start at low doses and increase slowly as some of its more dangerous side effects are dose-dependent. It should be given three times a day with total daily doses ranging from 200 mg to 800 mg, which is the maximum recommended daily dose.

Advantages and Disadvantages.   As could be assumed, thioridazine has more disadvantages than advantages. Its main potential advantage is that it can be tried when other antipsychotics have been unsuccessful. It is not considered a first-line medication but has been shown to be effective in some people who do not respond to other antipsychotics. Its disadvantages far outweigh its potential advantages. The population that this medication could be used for must be considered, as it could potentially be more dangerous in children and the elderly. One of its other disadvantages is its interactions with other medications, especially those that may also prolong the QT interval. One must be aware of what other medications a patient may be taking, as the cardiac interval prolongation can be additive with other medications and put the patient at much higher risk.

FDA-Approved Uses.   Thioridazine is only FDA-approved for one use; it is approved for treatment in schizophrenic patients who have failed to respond to other antipsychotic drugs. Its branded form, Mellaril, was voluntarily taken off the market by its producer because of concerns for toxicity to the heart and to the eyes. The generic form is still used occasionally but infrequently.

Off-Label Uses.   Low doses of it are commonly used in Russia for treatment of somatoform disorders, panic attacks, hyperactive and impulsive forms of ADHD, and insomnia related to alcohol withdrawal.

Mid Potency

The mid potency class of typical antipsychotics are probably the least discussed and least used class of antipsychotics. They again are classified according to their potency. Since they are mid potency, they will not be efficacious at a very low dose, but they will likely be efficacious at a dose lower than the low potency typicals. They have a similar side effect profile to the low potency typicals, but the anticholinergic and antihistaminic effects may not be as prominent, as the doses used are generally a little lower than the low potency class.

Perphenazine

Perphenazine is a phenothiazine derivative that has been used for decades in the United States as a treatment for psychosis. It is marketed in the United States as Trilafon. It is approximately five times as potent as chlorpromazine (low potency).

Therapeutics. Similar to previously mentioned antipsychotics, perphenazine's antipsychotic properties come from its ability to block dopamine receptors in the brain, leading to a decrease in psychotic symptoms. It also has some antihistaminic and anticholinergic effects. It works on cholinergic receptors in the vomiting center making it helpful to reduce nausea and vomiting in certain situations. If giving the pill form of this medication, it likely takes about one week to see improvement in psychotic symptoms and takes several weeks to show full effects on behavior. This medication is also available in an injectable form. When given by this route, the medication is injected directly into the muscle, similar to how vaccinations are given. If giving the medication by an injectable route, an initial effect can be seen within about 10 minutes, and the medication peaks at a few hours. If being used for nausea and vomiting, the results are generally rather immediate.

Side Effects. Similar to all other antipsychotics, because of the blocking of dopamine, this medication can cause movement side effects. Because of its action on histamine and acetylcholine, it can cause weight gain, sedation, blurred vision, constipation, and dry mouth. With this medication, the sedation is usually transient, and while sedation is a common side effect, it is not as notable as the sedation with the low potency antipsychotics.

Dosing and Usage. Perphenazine is available in tablet and injection formulations. It is given at different doses and different routes depending on whether the treatment is meant for psychotic symptoms or nausea and vomiting. For psychosis the general oral dose range is around 12–24 mg daily for patients living in the community and much higher for patients who are hospitalized (16–64 mg per day). As mentioned earlier, there is an injection formulation of perphenazine that can be used to treat psychosis. This is started at an initial dose of 5 mg and can be increased to a maximum of 15 mg per day. When treating nausea and vomiting, the route of medication can again be oral or injected into the muscle, and the dose is much lower. Generally the dose range is between 8 and 16 mg per day when taking the tablets and the treating dose with the muscle injection is 5 mg.

Advantages and Disadvantages. Not all of the antipsychotics are available to be injected into the muscle. This could be advantageous in emergency situations. Similarly, and partially because of its intramuscular form, it is a useful medication for patients with physical hyperactivity and violent or aggressive behavior (in the setting of other psychotic symptoms). As with other antipsychotics, it needs to be used with caution in certain age groups like the elderly and children. Perphenazine has been shown in large studies to have comparable effectiveness compared to the newer, atypical antipsychotics. And while it carries a similar side effect profile to the low potency antipsychotics, it is less likely to cause the sedation and decrease in blood pressure that the low potency medications cause.

FDA-Approved Uses. Perphenazine is approved by the FDA for two uses: schizophrenia and nausea and vomiting. For schizophrenia it is approved and can be used for emergent and immediate management of psychotic symptoms as well as continued use for long-term management. It is not used for general nausea and vomiting but only for severe symptoms in adults. While its risk during pregnancy cannot be ruled out, it is sometimes used during pregnancy for relief of violent nausea and vomiting. When being used to treat these symptoms, it is only used for short-term management.

Off-Label Uses. As far as psychotic symptoms and disorders, perphenazine is only approved for schizophrenia; however, it is used to treat various other psychotic disorders and symptoms. It is not approved for the acute manic episodes of bipolar disorder or the psychotic symptoms that go along with these episodes. It is sometimes used off-label to manage those symptoms in an acute manic phase but not generally used for continued maintenance treatment of bipolar disorder.

High Potency

The high potency antipsychotics have the strongest attraction to the dopamine receptors. Like the other typical antipsychotics, they work on the psychotic symptoms by blocking dopamine in the brain. Because they have the strongest attraction to the dopamine receptors, they are the most potent, meaning that the dose needed to see improvement in symptoms is relatively low compared to the other typical antipsychotics. Similar to the other typical antipsychotics, the high potency medications have some impact on acetylcholine and histamine leading to antihistaminic and anticholinergic side effects. However, since they require a relatively low dose, these side effects are less common and less severe when using the high potency medications. On the other hand, since they have such a strong attraction to the dopamine receptors, the movement side effects are more common when using the high potency medications. While in general the newer atypical antipsychotics are used more frequently for treatment, the high potency antipsychotics are still used quite frequently and can be very useful in certain populations and situations.

Haloperidol

Haloperidol is a butyrophenone derivative that works to treat psychotic symptoms by blocking dopamine receptors in the brain. Its generic name is haloperidol, and its marketed trade name is Haldol. It is a high potency antipsychotic, meaning it has a very strong attraction to the dopamine receptors. It actually is known to work on two different types of dopamine receptors in the brain leading it to relieve not only psychotic symptoms but also tics and other symptoms of Tourette's syndrome. It is currently on the WHO Model List of Essential Medicines—the medicines that are considered the most important medicines to the human health system.

Therapeutics. Haloperidol works on one dopamine pathway in the brain to block receptors and reduce many of the symptoms of psychosis, including some of the aggressive and explosive behaviors. It works on a different dopamine pathway in the brain to block receptors and improve some of the symptoms of Tourette's syndrome such as tics and vocal abnormalities. Improvement in symptoms can be seen within a few days, and some improvement is expected within one week; however, the full effect of the medication on symptoms may not be seen for several weeks.

Side Effects. As mentioned previously, the action taken on dopamine receptors in the brain is what is considered responsible for the reduction in psychotic symptoms. The action taken on various dopamine receptors in different pathways in the brain is also what is responsible for the movement side effects of various antipsychotics. Since haloperidol has such a strong attraction for dopamine receptors, it is more likely than other medications to cause some of these movement side effects. These side effects range in severity, and some of them are reversible if you stop the medication or decrease the dose. The reversible movement side effects include muscle rigidity and akathisia. Akathisia is often described as an internal feeling of restlessness that causes patients to have trouble being comfortable. They will often appear restless, moving from seated position to standing and pacing because they cannot find comfort. Patients taking haloperidol can also undergo a side effect called dystonia, which is a severe muscle rigidity often causing the patient pain. One of the classic presentations of this is a person who looks like he or she has his or her neck turned quite strongly to one side and is staring to the side. However, he or she is unable to move his or her neck and will complain of pain. This usually can be treated with an anticholinergic medication (like Benadryl) with nearly immediate results. Haloperidol has a strong attraction to dopamine receptors and a weaker attraction to other receptors like histamine and acetylcholine. Therefore, it still has the potential to

cause some of the side effects like sedation, weight gain, blurry vision, and constipation that low potency antipsychotics are more known for, but it is less common
in the high potency medications.

Dosing and Usage.   Haloperidol is quite diverse in its available routes of
administration. It is currently available in a tablet, liquid, muscular injection,
IV use, and a long-acting depot injection. If it is being used by either the tablet
or liquid route, its general dosing range is between 1 and 40 mg per day. The
maximum daily dose of oral haloperidol should be no greater than 100 mg.
If it is being used as an immediate-release injectable form, either injected
directly into the muscle or through an IV, then it is generally dosed somewhere
between 2 and 5 mg. This same dose can be repeated as often as every hour,
but the patient should be switched to an oral form as soon as possible. The
depot injection of haloperidol is slowly released over a period of time, and once
a patient is at a maintenance dose, he or she requires the medication only once
a month. When beginning a depot injection with a patient, the goal should be
10–20 times the daily dose that he or she was receiving orally.

Advantages and Disadvantages.   While haloperidol is a culprit for causing
some of the movement side effects that are not desirable, it does have some
characteristics that can make it quite advantageous. It is available in the injectable form that can be used in emergent and dangerous situations, meaning that
when a medication is needed to immediately diffuse a situation, it can prove to
be quite beneficial. It also has a long-acting depot form that can be very helpful
with patients who have trouble remembering to take their medications or do
not like taking their medications. There are a few other antipsychotics that
have a depot form as well. Haloperidol's depot form requires administration
only once a month, which can be quite convenient for some patients. Most
of the antipsychotics that have been discussed work on the positive symptoms
of psychosis. These were described earlier as the symptoms that are most
noticeable to the surrounding community; they include the hallucinations,
delusions, and disorganized behaviors. If a patient responds to a relatively
low dose of haloperidol (about 2–5 mg a day), it has been shown that he or
she may show improvement not only in the positive symptoms of the psychotic disorder but in the negative symptoms as well. This can be extremely
beneficial in helping patients become more productive and included members
of their community. Generally at those low doses, they are also less likely to
suffer from side effects. Haloperidol is an older medication as well, so while
it remains quite effective it is available at a very low cost. As with most other
antipsychotics, they can be harmful in certain populations, and special care

and consideration need to be taken into account before using haloperidol in children or the elderly. Since they are more prone to causing the movement disorder side effects, they need to be taken into consideration and discussed prior to starting this as a long-term treatment. While at lower doses haloperidol can improve some of the negative symptoms of psychotic disorders, at higher doses it can worsen cognitive function, which should be considered when choosing a treatment medication as well.

FDA-Approved Uses. Haloperidol has been relatively well studied and is approved for many different uses by the FDA. For psychosis it is approved for the long-term treatment of schizophrenia. It is approved for more immediate use in manifestations of psychotic disorders; this is where the intramuscular and IV forms of the medication would be used. As mentioned previously, because of its action on a different pathway of dopamine receptors, it has been shown to be beneficial in the treatment of Tourette's syndrome and is FDA-approved for that. It has been approved as a second-line treatment for some behaviors in children. Second-line treatment means that there are other medications that have a better risk/benefit ratio and should be tried first, but if they fail, haloperidol is approved for use. It is approved as second-line treatment of severe behavior problems of children with explosive and aggressive hyperexcitability. It is also approved as second-line treatment for short-term use in children with hyperactivity.

Off-Label Uses. Haloperidol has a number of FDA-approved uses but still is used as an off-label medication for certain disorders. As many of the antipsychotics already mentioned, haloperidol is used in the treatment of bipolar disorder, yet it has not been approved for this. This medication is often used to help control behavior in dementia; however, it is not FDA-approved for this and it is not risk-free in this population. The risks of using haloperidol (and other antipsychotics) in dementia will be discussed in further detail in following chapters. Haloperidol is also sometimes used in the treatment of delirium but has not been FDA-approved for this. People who become delirious, from some type of medical condition, often have psychotic symptoms that could be relieved with short-term use of an antipsychotic like haloperidol.

Fluphenazine

Fluphenazine is another high potency typical antipsychotic, marketed in the United States under the brand name of Prolixin. It is a phenothiazine derivative that improves psychotic symptoms by blocking dopamine in the brain.

Similar to haloperidol, it is a high potency medication, so it has a very strong attraction to the dopamine receptors.

Therapeutics. Fluphenazine blocks dopamine receptors in the brain and by that mechanism helps to reduce positive symptoms of psychosis. Once starting the medication and using it regularly, one should see improvement in psychotic symptoms within about one week. However, full effect on behaviors can take several weeks of regular medication use.

Side Effects. As a high potency antipsychotic, fluphenazine is more likely to cause some of the movement disorders than the low or mid potency medications. This is because, like haloperidol, fluphenazine has such a strong attraction to the dopamine receptors. These high potency antipsychotics are unable to select specific receptors that are involved only in psychotic symptoms. Instead, they end up generally blocking various dopamine receptors in different pathways. Therefore, they have a strong attraction to the dopamine receptors in the psychotic symptom pathways as well as the dopamine receptors in the movement pathways. Like haloperidol, this can lead to rigidity and akathisia, which are reversible. It can also lead to specific movements of the mouth and face over time, called tardive dyskinesia, which is not reversible. Also similar to haloperidol, fluphenazine can cause some of the same anticholinergic and antihistaminic side effects that are readily seen in low potency and mid potency medications. But these side effects are less common in fluphenazine as well as other high potency antipsychotics.

Dosing and Usage. Fluphenazine comes in many different forms of administration. It is available in a tablet, liquid, short-term immediate-release injectable form (to be given intramuscularly), and a long-acting decanoate injectable form. The general dosing and range of dosing vary depending on the type of administration being used. Again, overall, the dosing should be relatively lower when compared to the low potency and mid potency, since the attraction to the dopamine receptors is so much stronger in this high potency class. When using the oral route of administration, the patient should be started on 0.5–10 mg a day, usually divided into multiple doses daily. The medication should be titrated up until maximum effect is reached, going no higher than 40 mg daily. The average dose range for the oral route is between 1 and 20 mg daily. When using the short-term immediate-release intramuscular route, the initial dose should be 1.25 mg. The maximum daily dose is generally considered 10 mg a day. Fluphenazine also comes in a long-acting decanoate form, which is similar to the decanoate of haloperidol but has different dosing guidelines. The initial dose of fluphenazine decanoate should be between 12.5 and

25 mg. It is generally dosed to be given every two to four weeks, depending on the individual and his or her reaction to the medication. After giving an initial dose, the patient should be monitored for improvement in symptoms and side effects, and the following maintenance doses should be either increased or decreased based on the individual's needs.

Advantages and Disadvantages. Fluphenazine's strong attraction to dopamine receptors and various forms of administration give it a profile that makes it advantageous in certain situations. Because of its strong attraction to dopamine, it has fewer side effects caused by other receptor pathways, meaning it has less weight gain, changes in blood pressure, constipation, blurry vision, and sedation, making it more suitable for certain populations. Still when using antipsychotics in children or the elderly, one must take precautions and closely monitor for side effects. Like haloperidol, since fluphenazine comes in an immediate-release intramuscular form, it can be advantageous in emergent situations. It can be very helpful in situations where a patient's behavior is escalating and he or she is putting himself or herself and/or others at risk of injury. Fluphenazine also comes in the long-acting decanoate injection, which can be very beneficial in populations that have a history of medication noncompliance or in patients who are not interested in taking a pill every day. The long-acting decanoate form can be much more convenient for some people. One of the advantages of fluphenazine's decanoate form is that it has a relatively rapid onset of action compared to some of the other long-acting injectables.

FDA-Approved Uses. Like many of the other typical antipsychotics, fluphenazine is FDA-approved for psychotic disorders. It is approved for long-term and short-term immediate-acting use in psychotic disorders. While it does have the short-term immediate-acting intramuscular form, it is not approved for management of aggressive behavior but only approved for use in treating psychotic symptoms.

Off-Label Uses. Also like many other antipsychotics, it is not approved by the FDA for use in the acute manic phase of bipolar disorder. However, it is used as an off-label medication in the acute manic phase to treat psychotic symptoms.

The previous descriptions cover only a portion of the typical antipsychotics that have been used in the United States and around the world. However, they do cover medications from each of the different categories. While all of the medications in a specific category are not exactly the same, they do tend to have similar profiles. So if one has a general understanding of the characteristics of medications in a category, these can largely be applied to other medications in the same category. They will have similar dose ranges, similar efficacy profiles, and similar side effect profiles.

As mentioned previously, when discussing the development of the antipsychotics, there was continued research to try to develop better antipsychotics. Because while the advent of chlorpromazine was revolutionary, patients were showing improvement in symptoms but not complete resolution, and there was a whole host of unwanted side effects. As research continued, new antipsychotics were developed that were considered somewhat fundamentally different than the typical antipsychotics and therefore were called atypical antipsychotics.

ATYPICAL ANTIPSYCHOTICS: AS THE STORY CONTINUES ...

Atypical antipsychotics are slightly harder to categorize than the typical antipsychotics because they all have slightly different profiles. As a group, the major difference between typical antipsychotics and atypical antipsychotics is that the typicals block dopamine receptors in the brain to cause a reduction in psychotic symptoms, while the atypicals block dopamine as well as serotonin receptors in the brain. It was initially felt that the atypical antipsychotics had a safer side effect profile and were more efficacious. However, in the past decade, some of these beliefs have been called into question. As more is learned about the specific medications and how they act in the brain, there seems to be less and less of a distinction between the two classes. However, at this time, they are still divided into typical antipsychotics and atypical antipsychotics. And, largely because of the side effects from the typicals, atypical antipsychotics recommended as the first choice, and typicals are still considered a second choice if the atypical is not effective. Since the atypicals are not broken down into their own categories, it is more difficult to get a full understanding of them as a group, and instead one has to learn about each medication individually. In the following pages, a few of the many atypical antipsychotics will be reviewed in order to get an understanding of the group as a whole.

Clozapine

Clozapine was the first atypical antipsychotic to be developed. It was developed in the 1960s and introduced into the market in the early 1970s. It was taken off the market because it was found to have a life-threatening side effect that came from a decrease in white blood cells and because it did not seem to be linked to the movement side effects, which at the time were considered to be a marker of efficacy. It was later reintroduced to the U.S. market in the 1990s as Clozaril. Like haloperidol, clozapine is on the WHO Model List of Essential Medicines.

Therapeutics.   Clozapine is unique even among the atypical antipsychotics. It is known to block dopamine receptors as well as various serotonin receptors in the brain. Most of the atypical antipsychotics work by blocking both dopamine and serotonin. However, clozapine has been found to be effective in patients who do not respond to other typical or atypical antipsychotics; it is used to treat patients who are refractory to other medications. It is thought that clozapine actually interacts with more serotonin receptors and various other neurotransmitter receptors and that this is what makes it effective when other medications are not. However, these various mechanisms are not well understood. It is thought that clozapine's actions on serotonin receptors lead to increased dopamine in certain regions of the brain that are responsible for potentially showing improvement in the negative side effects, meaning that it leads to improvement in long-term cognition and improves a patient's ability to show emotion and interact with others.

Side Effects.   Most of the atypical antipsychotics have a higher risk of weight gain and sedation as side effects, and clozapine is no exception. Both can be problematic when taking clozapine and need to be closely monitored. Clozapine is well known for some relatively benign side effects and some life-threatening side effects. It is known to cause increased salivation, which while relatively benign, can be quite severe and bothersome for patients. It is also known to cause increased sweating. On the other side of the spectrum, it is known to be associated with many severe side effects and carries black box warnings for a number of them. It is well known for its association with agranulocytosis, which is a life-threatening lowering of white blood cells. People with agranulocytosis have a very low white blood cell count and are at very high risk for serious and dangerous infections. Because of this side effect, there are strict regulations and monitoring placed on the use of clozapine that will be discussed in later chapters. Clozapine has another black box warning for a specific disease of the heart called myocarditis. This disease causes an inflammation of the heart muscle. Some of the initial signs are fever and difficulty breathing. It can be monitored during treatment by checking some of the laboratory cardiac inflammation markers. Generally myocarditis is seen within the first month of initiating the medication, but it should not be forgotten as a possible side effect further along in treatment. Clozapine also has a black box warning for seizures as it has an increased risk of seizures as the dose increases. While clozapine has some dangerous side effects and the weight gain can be problematic, it does have the least association with the extrapyramidal movements associated with many of the antipsychotics.

Dosing and Usage.   Clozapine is only available in the United States to be taken orally. Since clozapine has many serious side effects, some of which are dependent on how high the dose is, there is strict monitoring in place, and all patients taking clozapine have to be registered in a clozapine database. There is a structured format for initiating the medication and titrating up the dose. The initial dose should be 12.5 mg two times a day. This dose can be increased by 25–50 mg each day until the desired effects are reached. General maintenance dosing is between 300 and 450 mg daily, with a maximum daily dose of 900 mg. If the medication needs to be discontinued, it should be slowly discontinued, decreasing by 100 mg a week or less. If clozapine is discontinued abruptly, a rebound psychosis can be seen with escalating psychotic symptoms.

Advantages and Disadvantages.   While clozapine has many disadvantages and needs to be used with precaution and special consideration in certain populations and not used at all in populations with certain diseases, it does have some great advantages that make it the best medication for certain groups. It should be used with caution in patients with kidney disease, liver disease, heart conditions, the elderly, children, and pregnant women. Since weight gain and increase in glucose and eventual diabetes are prevalent in those using clozapine, it should be used cautiously in people who are already overweight or have diabetes. One of clozapine's greatest advantages is that it has been shown to be effective in treating patients who have not responded to other antipsychotics. So in a population of people who have been refractory to other treatments, clozapine may be an excellent choice. Clozapine has also been shown to decrease suicide in patients with schizophrenia. So it could be advantageous to use in a population of patients with psychotic disorders (specifically schizophrenia and schizoaffective disorder) who show suicidal behaviors.

FDA-Approved Uses.   Clozapine is not approved as a first-line antipsychotic but is FDA-approved for treatment-resistant schizophrenia. Clozapine is one of two psychotropic medications that has been shown to decrease suicide (the other being lithium). It is FDA-approved for use to reduce risk of recurrent suicidal behavior in patients with schizophrenia or schizoaffective disorder.

Off-Label Uses.   Since clozapine has so many serious side effects and is regulated and monitored so closely, it does not have many off-label uses. All of its off-label uses are also not first-line uses, but it is used when other medications have failed. It has been used in the treatment of bipolar disorder when patients have failed the FDA-approved medications. It has also been used in violent and aggressive patients with psychosis and other brain disorders, such as traumatic brain injury, when they have not responded to the FDA-approved treatments for those disorders.

Risperidone

After clozapine was reintroduced in the 1990s, it was a huge success, and this success furthered the desire to develop more antipsychotics that had a similar profile, specifically meaning that they did not cause the movement side effects and they showed some improvement in the negative symptoms of schizophrenia. Risperidone was the next developed and was approved in 1994 and is marketed as Risperdal. Risperidone is another antipsychotic on the WHO Model List of Essential Medicines.

Therapeutics.   Risperidone is structurally based on haloperidol with some changes. It, like the other atypical antipsychotics, works on multiple receptors in the brain; most notably it blocks dopamine and serotonin. Many of the atypical antipsychotics work on both dopamine and serotonin. However, both dopamine and serotonin have multiple different pathways and various subcategories of receptors. It is thought that the different atypicals likely work on different subcategories of serotonin and that may give them their more specific efficacy profiles. For instance, it is thought that risperidone works on a specific serotonin subcategory that makes it somewhat helpful in depression. These more specific pathways and receptors will be discussed in more detail in the chapter focused on explaining how antipsychotics work at a chemical level.

Side Effects.   Like the other antipsychotics, while it is felt that the therapeutic aspect comes from its work on blocking dopamine and serotonin, it also has effects on other types of neurotransmitters, like histamine, that lead to some side effects. It is common to see weight gain and sedation with risperidone use. While it is less likely to see movement side effects with risperidone and other atypical antipsychotics, it remains a side effect to be aware of.

Dosing and Usage.   Risperidone is available in oral and injectable forms. In the oral form, it can be given as a tablet or a liquid. It is generally started at 0.5 mg two times a day in a nonemergent adult situation. If the patient is in a more emergent psychotic state, perhaps requiring hospitalization, risperidone is started at a higher daily dose. It is generally increased by about 1 mg per day, until the desired results are seen. The maximum daily dose is considered to be 16 mg; however, the general dose range for healthy adults is between 2 and 8 mg per day. Risperidone can be used in the elderly and children and generally is dosed between 0.5 and 2 mg per day orally. Risperidone is also available in a long-acting intramuscular form. The long-acting form comes in doses ranging from 12.5 to 50 mg. Unlike some of the typical antipsychotics, risperidone has to be given every two weeks. However, it is still more desirable to some to get an injection once every two weeks as opposed to taking a medication every day.

Advantages and Disadvantages.   Because of the way that risperidone is processed by the body, it needs to be used with caution in patients with kidney problems and liver problems. It can still be used in these populations, but there are further guidelines to consider when dosing to ensure proper clearance of the medication and to avoid any further damage. Risperidone is actually FDA-approved for treatment in some children and adolescents, but the dosing is different than for a healthy adult. Risperidone is also one of the antipsychotics that is well accepted for treating agitation in the elderly with dementia. So while it is important to be cautious when dealing with these more sensitive populations, it may be advantageous to use.

FDA-Approved Uses.   Risperidone is approved by the FDA for a number of uses. It is approved for use in psychotic disorders. More specifically, it has been approved for use in schizophrenia for patients as young as 13. It is one of the antipsychotics that has been FDA-approved for the treatment of bipolar disorder and is actually approved for use in acute manic episodes for patients aged 10 and older. But it has also been approved for maintenance treatment of bipolar disorder. For these situations it can be used either with another mood-stabilizing medication or can be used as the sole treatment. Lastly, it has been approved for autism-related irritability in children aged 5 to 16.

Off-Label Uses.   While risperidone is FDA-approved for a number of uses, there are still some instances where it is used as an off-label medication. While it is generally well accepted to be used in the elderly with dementia to treat agitation, it is not FDA-approved for the treatment of any behavioral disturbances, no matter what the age of the patient. It has been noted to have some antidepressant qualities and so is sometimes used to treat bipolar depression; however, it is only approved to treat mania and for maintenance medication once stabilized.

Quetiapine

Quetiapine is another atypical antipsychotic that was developed in the 1990s and was approved by the FDA in 1997. It is most commonly marketed as Seroquel. Clozapine was looked upon as extremely effective but somewhat dangerous because of its side effect profile. Because of this, researchers wanted to develop drugs similar to clozapine with the hopes that they could be somewhat altered to change the side effects and keep the therapeutic effects. Quetiapine was the outcome and was developed as a derivation of clozapine.

Therapeutics. Like the other atypical antipsychotics, quetiapine's therapeutic benefit comes from its action at multiple different receptor sites, most notably dopamine and serotonin. It serves as a blockade at both dopamine and serotonin receptors. It is thought, especially since quetiapine is derived from clozapine, that it has effect at a number of other receptor sites and that this may be why it has been found to be effective in some treatment-resistant depression or bipolar depression. It is thought that the specific subcategory of serotonin receptor that quetiapine blocks plays a role in its ability to be effective in some treatment-resistant patients as well as why it has been shown to be helpful in improving patients' cognition and ability to emotionally relate to others.

Side Effects. One of quetiapine's most notable side effects is sedation. It is known to be more frequent and more significant in quetiapine when compared to other antipsychotics. For this reason, it is often given at nighttime. Quetiapine is also known for causing decreases in blood pressure upon standing (called orthostatic hypotension), which needs to be considered when using this medication in the elderly and is another reason it is often dosed at nighttime. Like the other atypical antipsychotics, quetiapine can cause weight gain with increases in cholesterol and blood sugar levels.

Dosing and Usage. Quetiapine is only available in oral forms, but unlike any of the previously mentioned antipsychotics, it comes in a regular tablet and an extended-release tablet. The difference between the regular tablet and extended-release tablet is simply in how many times the medication is given throughout the day. It is dosed two times a day for the regular tablet and once a day if giving the extended-release. Generally it is started at around 100 mg per day with a maximum approved daily dose of 800 mg. The usual dose range is between 400 and 800 mg for schizophrenia and mania and 300 mg for bipolar depression.

Advantages and Disadvantages. Like many other antipsychotics, quetia-pine can be used, rather should be used, with caution in the elderly and children, often requiring lower doses than in healthy adults. Quetiapine is thought to have a slower onset of improvement in symptoms, so it may not be a wise choice in a patient who needs emergent/urgent onset of action. As mentioned previously, quetiapine is known, more than other antipsychotics, for its sedation. This is more notable in some patients than others but may not be the best choice for a patient who has trouble tolerating sedation. Many of the antipsychotics are known to worsen symptoms in patients with Parkinson's disease and Lewy body dementia. However, quetiapine is not known to do that and may be the preferred choice for a patient with Parkinson's or Lewy body who needs an antipsychotic or a mood stabilizer. Quetiapine can be used in bipolar depression, which most antipsychotics are not approved for. It has also been found to be useful in situations where the patient has tried multiple medications and had poor results, similar to clozapine.

FDA-Approved Uses. Quetiapine also has a number of FDA approvals that might make it more advantageous in certain situations. It is approved for schizophrenia in adults and children as young as 13. It is also approved for acute manic episodes in adults and children as young as 10. Quetiapine has a wide range of approval for bipolar disorder. It is approved for the acute manic state, long-term maintenance, and bipolar depression. Unlike many of the other antipsychotics, it is also approved for unipolar depression (known simply as depression).

Off-Label Uses. Overall, quetiapine, which is derived from clozapine, has a relatively benign side effect profile with many of the benefits that clozapine has, and, therefore, it has many approved uses and is used as an off-label medication frequently. It is often used off-label for the treatment of agitation in patients with dementia, specifically Parkinson's disease and Lewy body dementia. Likely, partly due to its sedating properties, it has been used to treat behavioral disturbances in children and adolescents. It is used in low doses for insomnia (again, because of its sedation), however, this is not an approved use.

Aripiprazole

Aripiprazole is an atypical antipsychotic that was approved by the FDA in 2002 and is marketed as Abilify.

Therapeutics. Like the other atypical antipsychotics, it is considered to work on multiple receptors, including dopamine and serotonin. Aripiprazole stands out from the other atypicals because while it does block some dopamine in the brain, it actually binds to some dopamine receptors to increase their activity. Theoretically, aripiprazole can increase dopamine in the areas needed to decrease the positive psychotic symptoms and decrease dopamine in the areas needed to improve cognition and negative symptoms. Aripiprazole also works on various subcategories of serotonin, which is why it is thought to be a good antidepressant as well.

Side Effects. Unlike many of the atypical and some typical antipsychotics, aripiprazole is known for having little weight gain or sedation as side effects. More than other antipsychotics it is actually known to be activating in some patients. It causes patients to feel restless (akathisia) more than other antipsychotics. And while some antipsychotics can be used to treat nausea and vomiting, aripiprazole can actually cause nausea and vomiting.

Dosing and Usage. Aripiprazole comes in a variety of routes of administration. It is available in an oral tablet or liquid form, in an immediate-release intramuscular injection, and a long-acting intramuscular injection. Aripiprazole has varying average doses for the different disorders it is used to treat and the different types of administration. When used to treat schizophrenia or mania, the average daily dose is between 15 and 30 mg a day. It can be used as an additional medication to augment an antidepressant in depression and then the dose is much lower, with the average between 2 and 10 mg a day. The long-acting injectable form is either dosed at 300 mg or 400 mg and is given once every four weeks.

Advantages and Disadvantages. Aripiprazole shares some of its profile with many of the other antipsychotics and therefore must be used with caution in the elderly and children. However, it is one of the antipsychotics that is approved for some treatment in children. It also has a few characteristics that separate it from many other antipsychotics making it advantageous in certain situations and populations. It has been shown to be beneficial in some cases of refractory psychosis, especially in bipolar disorder. It is thought to have a low risk of weight gain compared to many of the other antipsychotics, so it should be considered when a patient is already overweight or has diabetes. It could also be advantageous to use in patients who do not tolerate sedation well as it can actually be activating.

FDA-Approved Uses. Likely, partly due to its somewhat unique profile, aripiprazole has FDA approval for a number of uses. It is approved for the treatment of schizophrenia in patients aged 13 and older. Aripiprazole is one of the antipsychotics that has approval for treatment in bipolar disorder. It is approved for the acute manic state for ages 10 and older, and it is approved as a maintenance treatment for bipolar disorder. Unlike many of the other antipsychotics, it has FDA approval for treatment of depression. It is not approved to be the sole treatment but is approved to be an add-on treatment for patients who do not completely respond to one of the first-line antidepressants. It is also FDA-approved for treatment of autism-related aggression in children aged 6–17.

Off-Label Uses.   Compared to some of the other antipsychotics, aripiprazole has a generally benign side effect profile and therefore is used on-label and off-label frequently. It is not approved for the treatment of bipolar depression but is used off-label. Aripiprazole, while not sedating and sometimes activating, can be effective in management of behavioral disturbances and is used off-label to treat disturbances in patients with dementia and children and adolescents.

Antipsychotics are a complicated group of medications that are difficult to categorize and are continuing to evolve with ongoing research prompted by the need for better medications. This chapter has provided a brief introduction to the group of medications as a whole—beginning with an understanding of the symptoms being treated, traveling through a discussion of the development of various treatments for psychosis, and ending with an examination of some of the individual medications. This chapter is meant to be a general overview, and the following chapters will delve into specific aspects of antipsychotics in greater detail. They will examine the history of their development, discuss exactly how they cause the effects and side effects that they do, how they are viewed in society, how they are regulated, and what the future holds for them.

Chapter 3

Antipsychotics: A Brief History

Serious mental illness has been a part of humanity since our most ancient roots. Each civilization had its own descriptions and belief about the causes of mental illness and potential remedies. Most theories focused on spiritual and religious disturbances.

Ancient Egyptians documented emotional distress and the inability to concentrate. They associated mental illness with dysfunction of the heart and mind and sought to treat the disorders with healing fluids, reciting chants, and taking the afflicted to religious temples. Ancient Hindu societies incorporated supernatural beliefs into their interpretations of mental disorders. As early as 600 BC, as part of the Hindu Ayurveda, an ancient medical text, the *Charaka Samhita*, hypothesized that mental illness was due to an imbalance in body fluids. The idea that illness was caused by a disturbance in the basic fluids, or *humors*, remained part of the medical dialogue for millennia. Treatments outlined included herbs, prayers, and use of charms or symbols. Ancient Chinese healers used acupuncture for mental illness, which is still practiced globally today. Ancient Greeks wrote extensively about mental illness. Some of the most recognized thinkers, including Socrates and Pythagoras, described experiencing auditory hallucinations, a classic feature of psychosis. Treatments were varied and included bloodletting, exorcism, physical restraint, beatings, starvation, and scaring the patient suddenly. The Old Testament refers often to mental illness and suggests that disorders are caused by a weak relationship between the patient and God.

In the modern era, originally in Europe, many people with symptoms that we would now recognize as part of a mental illness, including hallucinations, delusions, and manic symptoms, were accused of being witches or other nonhuman entities. As such, many people with mental illnesses were punished or put to death. There were tribunals to establish if a person was a witch or merely insane. The insane were sent to jails or "madhouses," which was certainly a bad fate but much better than the one that awaited those judged to be witches.

The earliest psychiatric hospitals existed in the Muslim world, likely influenced by the Quranic verse, "Do not give the property with which God has entrusted you to the insane, but feed and clothe them with this property and speak kindly to them." The first hospital was built in Baghdad in 705 AD, followed by others in Cairo and Damascus.

The oldest psychiatric hospital in Europe was the Bethlem Royal Hospital in London, which began serving the mentally ill in the 13th and 14th centuries. However, the notion of the traditional psychiatric asylum as a way to address the problem of mental illness did not gain popularity in Europe until the 19th century. A series of important laws in England and France funded these institutions and later regulated them as abuses were reported. In general, as mentioned elsewhere in this text, the function of these asylums was not necessarily to treat the patients. They were established to treat society by removing the burden that the mentally ill represented. As the focus of the economy shifted from agriculture to industry and people began to move from the country to the city, people were living in closer quarters. Therefore, the disorganized behavior of the mentally ill was a bigger problem. Conditions at these asylums were often inhumane. However, there were significant movements at the time to improve the conditions of the asylums and limit the abuses. French psychiatrist and reformer Philippe Pinel removed inhumane methods of physical restraints, like chain and other devices, from his hospitals in the 19th century.

Pennsylvania Hospital in Philadelphia was the first hospital in the United States to treat patients with mental illness. While it was mostly used for medical conditions, the basement had rooms that were equipped with shackles and other restraining instruments. The first hospital built entirely for the treatment of the mentally ill was Eastern State Hospital in Williamsburg, Virginia, in 1773.

Throughout the 19th and early 20th centuries, psychiatric hospitals were constructed throughout the country. Most of these facilities were public, as people with serious mental illnesses rarely had the resources to afford private hospitalizations. Further, as the populations of urban centers expanded, the government appreciated the potential dangers of untreated mental illnesses and needed more availability of treating institutions. Because agitation and disorganized behavior are common symptoms of schizophrenia and other psychotic illnesses, the environment of the hospitals was dangerous and unsanitary. Furthermore, these hospitals were generally underfunded. Due to the stigma of mental illness at the time, hospitalized patients did not have a substantial lobby advocating for adequate conditions.

EARLY BIOLOGIC REMEDIES: THE ORIGINAL ANTIPSYCHOTICS

Toward the beginning of the 20th century, scientists in the United States began hypothesizing about the biological causes of mental illness and experimenting with potential treatments. While their intentions were sound, the poor understanding of the mental illness and the catastrophic results of their actions did more harm than good. In retrospect, their actions appear barbaric. However, they represented the best attempts of contemporary physicians to address difficult medical problems.

One hypothesis in the early 20th century attributed serious mental illness to an infection in the brain. We now know that this hypothesis is wrong, but it was not a terrible thought. In general, infections in any body system cause dysfunction. A viral or bacterial infection of the gastrointestinal system (gastroenteritis) causes dysfunction in the form of nausea, vomiting, and diarrhea. A viral or bacterial infection in the male reproductive system (orchitis) can cause dysfunction in the form of sterility. So why should not a brain infection lead to schizophrenia? Furthermore, known cases of infection in the central nervous system, which involves the brain and spinal cord (meningitis), involve cognitive changes. Patients with meningitis often become confused, irritable, and drowsy. At the time when this hypothesis was popular, antibiotics, which are now the standard treatment of bacterial infections, had not been synthesized. So, in order to treat mentally ill patients of their "infection," doctors developed an unusual method. To kill the bacteria, they induced a fever in mentally ill patients by transfusing blood infected with malaria. Malaria is a parasitic illness common in tropical climates that is known to cause high fevers, sometimes up to 105 degrees F. For years physicians "treated" mental illness this way, and while they successfully induced high fevers, illnesses like schizophrenia never resolved because the hypothesis was incorrect. Instead of curing mental illness, doctors just spread malaria. After this treatment failed enough times and was clearly shown to be not worth the risk, the practice of infected blood transfusion ended. However, the pioneer of the field, Austrian psychiatrist Julius Wagner Jauregg, was awarded a Nobel Prize in Medicine for his work.

Another type of medical therapy was developed from the same incorrect infectious hypothesis of serious mental illness. Some physicians believed mental illness was caused by bacteria involved in tooth infections that spread to the brain. This assumption was made because many patients with schizophrenia and other serious mental illnesses have poor dentition and often lose their teeth by adulthood. Therefore, the intervention that some physicians made was to remove all the teeth of patients as soon as schizophrenia was identified. This would presumably prevent future tooth infections and limit the infectious process that they believed exacerbated or perpetuated mental illness. However, because the infection hypothesis was incorrect, this treatment was no more successful than the malaria blood transfusions. No mental illness was cured, and patients needlessly suffered incredibly painful dental surgeries and then lived their lives without teeth. The reason many patients with schizophrenia had and continue to have poor dentition is because the disorganization that is a hallmark of the illness makes it difficult to consistently plan and execute routine tasks, like brushing teeth and following up with a dentist.

Later, physicians believed that mental illness resulted from an overactive mind. Therefore, various methods were utilized to slow down brain activity. This was first achieved by submerging patients with mental illness in "cold water baths." Patients were wrapped in nearly freezing towels, and their core body temperature was decreased (hypothermia), sometimes to the point of causing a comatose state. Patients were then brought back to normal temperatures.

Another method of slowing down brain activity in patients with mental illness was with the administration of excessive amounts of insulin. Insulin is a hormone produced by the pancreas that facilitates the influx of glucose from the blood into the cells of the body. If too much insulin is given, blood glucose becomes dangerously low (hypoglycemia). The brain is powered by blood glucose, so after insulin overdoses, it is no longer able to function efficiently and patients become comatose. Occasionally diabetic patients take too much insulin and their blood glucose becomes too low, but there are warning signs, such as dizziness, fatigue, and clammy hands. Properly educated diabetic patients know how to quickly find some candy or orange juice to regulate their glucose levels.

Another Austrian psychiatrist named Manfred Sakel used insulin to treat patients who were addicted to morphine, a commonly abused opioid at the time. He noticed that insulin administration had a calming effect on patients who were in the unpleasant state of withdrawal. He began to institute a regimen of insulin-induced hypoglycemic comas. Patients were often kept in the coma for several hours and then revived with injections of glucose. This was repeated five days a week, for several weeks. It proved dangerous, with a mortality rate of between 5 and 10 percent.

When hypothermic or hypoglycemic mentally ill patients were restored to a baseline physiology, they would occasionally show cognitive impairment or slowing that might imply a treatment of symptoms. For example, if a psychotic patient was screaming because he or she was under the paranoid delusional belief that an assassin was targeting him or her and he or she was put into a coma with freezing cold temperatures or hypoglycemia, he or she would probably not resume the same state of psychotic panic immediately upon regaining consciousness. His brain functioning would be slower and he would move slower, talk slower, and think slower. However, after enough time, when his brain would recover, the mental illness would be back to baseline levels. Therefore, after enough trials, these interventions, and the hypotheses behind them, were debunked.

Electroconvulsive therapy (ECT) was also a mainstream treatment of serious mental illnesses. It was frequently used in the state hospital system in the 1940s. ECT was based on two scientific innovations. The first was the observation, which later turned out to be false, that patients with epilepsy (an illness that involves regular seizures) had a reduced incidence of mental illness. The other discovery was that seizures could be induced by passing electrical current through the brain. Two Italian physicians induced seizures in animals by connecting them to electrodes. Psychiatrists connected these two principles and administered serial ECT treatments to hospitalized patients. After more research, it was shown that ECT was not effective in treating schizophrenia but was useful in patients with severe depression and catatonia, a psychiatric problem manifested by an inability to move. Early practitioners of ECT often did not use appropriate anesthesia and muscle relaxants, so some patients were physically injured due to the convulsions. Due to certain media reports and movies like *One Flew over the Cuckoo's Nest*, which portrayed ECT delivered with abusive and punitive methods, ECT fell out of favor among the public. ECT became a highly stigmatized treatment that patients generally do not want, so physicians do not offer as much as may be clinically indicated. However, it is still used today and remains the most effective treatment for patients with severe mood disorders. It is no longer relevant as an antipsychotic intervention.

In the late 1930s, another procedure emerged in the treatment of serious mental illness called the lobotomy. Although various types of psychosurgeries had been attempted beginning in the late 19th century, this was the most infamous and commonly performed procedure. The lobotomy was a drastic method to control symptoms, and it was implemented in ways that horrendously abused the civil liberties of patients with mental illness. In many ways, psychiatry as a field has yet to recover from the public relations crisis that transpired when the American public realized what the lobotomy was and how it was being performed.

The lobotomy was developed by the Portuguese neurologist, and later politician, Antonio Egas Moniz. He believed that there was an organic basis for mental illness, and it was rooted in the connections between different areas of the brain. Therefore, he postulated that severing these connections could address symptoms. The first leucotomy, as he called the procedure, was performed in Lisbon on November 12, 1935. The patient was put under general anesthesia, and several holes were drilled through the skull. Ethanol was then injected along the tracts that connected the frontal lobe with other areas of the brain, which rendered them dysfunctional. The goal, therefore, was to create what Moniz called a "frontal barrier," cutting off the frontal lobe from the rest of the brain. Later, he and his colleagues began using a surgical device to sever the tracts. When he published the reports of his first 20 cases, he reported that 35% showed significant improvement, 35% showed some improvement, and 30% were unchanged. He reported that no patients died during the procedure and downplayed adverse outcomes such as urinary incontinence, autonomic dysregulation, apathy, visual problems, and lethargy. Several of his colleagues criticized Moniz' procedure, including the physician who cared for the patients after they returned to the hospital. The treating physician noted them to have diminished personalities. Nevertheless, Moniz continued to travel throughout Europe and demonstrate the leucotomy to physicians. Many countries, including England and Italy, had centers that regularly performed the surgery.

In 1937, an Italian physician named Amarro Fiamberti innovated the procedure to make it less dangerous and intrusive. Instead of boring holes through patient's skulls, Fiamberti was able to access the connections between the frontal orbit and other parts of the part through the orbit, the part of the skull that creates the eye socket. This improvement had a profound impact on the American neuropsychiatrist Walter Freeman.

As medical director of St. Elizabeth's Hospital in Washington, DC, Freeman extensively researched the causes of mental illness. He met Moniz at a conference, and Moniz encouraged him to practice leucotomies in the United States. Freeman performed America's first leucotomy in 1936. The following year he published a manual on a variation of Moniz' technique and renamed the procedure the "lobotomy." He continued to amend the surgery. The major problem he saw was that the operation involved too many resources to be widely utilized. It required a surgeon, an anesthesiologist, general anesthesia, and an operating room. Therefore, it was not a practical way to treat the hundreds of thousands of mentally ill patients in the state hospitals. In 1945, Freeman began experimenting with an ice pick he found in his home. Working with cadavers, he developed a way to force the ice pick through the orbit with a mallet and sever the fibers that connect regions of the brain.

Freeman began performing the "icepick lobotomy" in 1946. Instead of general anesthesia, patients were induced to developed seizures by ECT. Therefore, the procedure could be accomplished outside of an operating room. Freeman marketed his "icepick lobotomy" extensively. He spoke at conferences, medical schools, and state hospitals. Large state hospitals were eager to allow Freeman to perform his operation as they were large, understaffed, and poorly equipped to properly manage the psychiatric needs of their patients. Freeman bought a van, named it the "lobotomobile," and travelled across the country, both operating and teaching the procedure. Up to 40,000 people in the United States received lobotomies, many performed either by Freeman or physicians he instructed.

Freeman's most famous patient was Rosemary Kennedy, President John F. Kennedy's sister. He operated on her in 1941 when Rosemary was 23. Rosemary had an intellectual disability, with an estimated IQ between 60 and 70. She had difficulty learning and was easily frustrated. As she got older, Rosemary suffered severe mood swings and behavior problems. Her father, Joseph Kennedy Sr., contacted Freeman and arranged the procedure. While many patients who received lobotomies had a psychotic disorder, like schizophrenia, Rosemary did not. Unfortunately, the procedure had poor results, as many of them did. She lost significant cognitive abilities, was unable to care for herself, and spent the rest of her life institutionalized in Wisconsin.

Freeman's work was widely criticized. In 1951, while posing for a picture during an operation in Iowa, he inadvertently knocked surgical instrument too far into the patient's brain, who later died. Freeman operated on several minors, the youngest of whom was four years old. He was eventually banned from performing the surgery in 1967 after his last patient died of a cerebral hemorrhage. However, he continued to practice medicine and fared better than his mentor Moniz, who was shot by a former patient in 1949.

"A DRUG IN SEARCH OF AN ILLNESS": DEVELOPING ANTIPSYCHOTIC MEDICATIONS

Like so many important scientific discoveries, antipsychotic medications were discovered in the search for something else. Between the middle of the 19th and 20th centuries, chemists developed the precursors to antipsychotics while trying to find solutions to problems like malaria and the lack of safe anesthesia during surgery. But even before that, chemists isolated the original ancestors of antipsychotics working in the textile and dye industry.

In 1856, a British scientist named W. H. Perkin was doing experiments to identify dyes. He created an artificial purple color, and in 1868, German chemists named Carl Grabe and Carl Liebermann produced a dye called aliza-rin from coal tar. In 1876, more experiments were done on previous chemists' work, which led to a dye called methylene blue. In 1883, August Bernthsen isolated a derivative compound called phenothiazine that would completely change the way the world understood and treated serious mental illnesses.

The first half of the 20th century was dominated by the two world wars. Malaria, a parasitic illness characterized by high fever, posed an enormous problem for armies traveling to tropical environments, on both sides of the conflicts. The typical treatment for malaria, quinine, derived from the bark of the *quina cinchona*, was not easily accessible to the troops. Scientists believed phenothiazine could be effective, but experiments did not show favor-able results.

Despite the phenothiazine's lack of antimalarial efficacy, researchers at one French laboratory called Rhone-Poulenc in Vitry-sur-Seine continued to search for potential uses. The lead researcher, Paul Charpentier, looked at the antihistaminergic properties of this class of drugs. They manipulated phe-nothiazine, adding different groups of atoms to parts of the chemical com-pound, and synthesized potent antihistamine called promethazine in the late 1940s.

Antihistamines had, and continue to have, many uses in medicine. They are the main treatment for allergies. In an allergic reaction, the allergen (particles of a peanut for example) interacts with a type of white blood cell called a mast cell, which stores histamine. When the allergen binds to the mast cell, hista-mine is released into the body, causing an allergic reaction, which can involve hives, sneezing, watery eyes, and, most seriously, swelling in parts of the respira-tory system, making it difficult to breathe. Antihistamines, as the name implies, block histamine and prevent or decrease the intensity of the allergic reaction. A Swiss scientist named Daniel Bouvet was an expert in allergies and was looking at promethazine exactly for this purpose at the same laboratory in France. Diphenhydramine, known better by its trade name, Benadryl, was developed out of this research and is now universally administered.

Antihistamines were also investigated for their potential role in surgical anesthesia. Because anesthesia was not as effective and reliable as it is today, undergoing surgery was an extremely stressful event, both physically and emo-tionally. Surgeons of the era described "surgical shock" as the body's desperate fight against the operation, which often led to slower recovery and emotional consequences. Now, this type of shock or physiologic distress is attributed to blood loss during surgery, but physicians of the day believed the shock was caused by dysfunction of the central nervous system. A French surgeon named Henri-Marie Laborit looked for a drug to prevent the body from triggering this stress response. He tried several medications with mixed results, before arriving at the newly synthesized promethazine. Laborit observed that when he combined promethazine with barbituates, which were given to put patients to sleep, the sedative effects lasted longer. He then combined barbituates, promethazine, and dolantine, which was an early narcotic painkiller, and created what became known as the "lytic cocktail." Laborit believed that the overstimulation of the nervous system leading to shock was caused by certain chemicals, such as histamine. He hypothesized that this combination of drugs would break or "lyse" the dangerous chemicals in the body, hence "lytic cocktail."

In addition to assisting with the sedating effects of anesthesia, promethazine and similar derivatives were noted to make the whole process of surgery—before, during, and after the operation—less traumatic. Patients given these medications, which included the precursors to antipsychotics, were less distressed by the process and more calm and therefore were noted to recover faster.

Due to the initial excitement over the potential for promethazine, scientists began experimenting with other similar compounds. One of those drugs was chlorpromazine, the first antipsychotic developed in December 1950. Chlorpromazine, now known by the trade name Thorazine, was found to have several interesting effects on animals. Scientists found that chlorpromazine extended the length of time dogs slept after they were given barbituates, which was important for surgery. It also decreased nausea and vomiting that dogs often experienced after they were given morphine, a powerful painkiller. A third discovery, and the one that foreshadowed its use in psychiatry, was that rats given chlorpromazine had a decreased conditioned avoidance reaction. Rats were taught or "conditioned" to associate a specific sound with an electric shock. Therefore, whenever the rats heard this sound, they immediately climbed a rope to avoid the shock, even long after the shock was not given. Rats given chlorpromazine were able to dissociate the sound from the shock and did not have the "conditioned response" of climbing the rope that other rats showed. That means that rats that were given the drug did not seem as distressed by the shocks as other rats. They were calmer and less able to be agitated and frightened.

In 1951, chlorpromazine was first used in humans. Patients were more able to tolerate the physical and emotional stress of surgery. Patients were generally more sedated and passive. Because of the observed calming effects of the medication, scientists passed along chlorpromazine to a group of professionals they thought might be able to make good use of it: psychiatrists. Laborit's intentions of revolutionizing surgery with these compounds ultimately failed.

The use of the central nervous depressants, in addition to other methods he used, like lowering surgical patients' temperatures with ice, led to an exacerbation of the surgical shock, as opposed to its cure. However, his decision to introduce his compounds to psychiatrists secured his legacy in the history of medicine.

The medication was given to psychiatrists at two hospitals in Paris, the Central Military Hospital and the Sainte-Anne Hospital. Psychiatrists at the Central Military Hospital first used chlorpromazine on a 57-year-old with bizarre and unpredictable behavior. He was admitted to the hospital after having assaulted others, exhibited grandiose behavior by making inappropriate political speeches in public, and walked around town professing his love of life. He was prescribed chlorpromazine, made significant improvements, and was able to be discharged in three weeks. In 1952, Laborit convinced psychiatrists to give chlorpromazine to an extremely manic 24-year-old patient known as Jacques Lh. Psychiatrists were shocked to see that he became calm and was able to resume his normal hospital activities and even play bridge. He was also discharged from the hospital in several weeks.

Jean Delay and Pierre Deniker, psychiatrists working at Sainte-Anne Hospital, are best known for adopting the practice of prescribing antipsychotics to psychiatric patients. Delay was the chairman of Department of Psychiatry at the University of Paris and had considerable influence on the field at the time. Delay knew Laborit personally and followed his research. Laborit was originally trained as a neurologist and had previously spent much of his career searching for medical and physical treatment for mental illness. The two began prescribing it with regularity in the hospitals and were able to notice effects within a more significant patient sample. Delay, Deniker, Laborit, and Heinz Lehmann, a Canadian psychiatrist who introduced chlorpromazine to North America, shared the prestigious Lasker Award in 1957. The award read: "For the introduction of chlorpromazine into psychiatry and for the demonstration that a medication can influence the clinical course of the major psychoses."

As discussed, antipsychotics were developed through a bizarre and unusual method. Usually, a problem leads to a discovery. In medicine, an illness may impact so many people, scientists are recruited to solve a public problem and find a cure. In this case, however, the precursors to antipsychotics were floating around for decades, essentially waiting for scientists to put them to the right use. For this reason, chlorpromazine has been called "a drug in search of an illness."

CHLORPROMAZINE RISES

In 1952, chlorpromazine was first marketed by the French pharmaceutical company Rhone-Poulenc as Largactil, which roughly means "large activity."

In 1954, the pharmaceutical firm Smith, Kline and French released chlorpromazine under the name Thorazine, as it is still known and used today. As the majority of the chemical development and first clinical trials of chlorpromazine took place in France, French psychiatrists, specifically in Paris and Lyons, were the first practitioners to incorporate antipsychotics as a main treatment of psychosis. They were eager to introduce it in their hospitals, mostly because their other treatments were ineffective and largely unhelpful.

Within several years, other European countries heard news of the French innovations and sought to replicate their success. In 1953, psychiatrists at Friedmatt Hospital in Basel, Switzerland, sent a colleague to the Sainte-Anne Hospital in Paris, the center of chlorpromazine treatment at the time, to take notes and report back. Soon after he told members of his department about chlorpromazine, it was widely administered to patients in the clinic. They evaluated the efficacy of chlorpromazine and found that up 48% of patients with psychosis for one to five years improved with chlorpromazine. No other therapy had achieved nearly that level of success. The medication was less successful with patients whose mental illness had been present for more than five years but was still far more effective than anything else at psychiatrists' disposal. The Swiss team may have been the first to realize that long-term psychosis is harder to treat, but this is a phenomenon that is well known to psychiatrists. Psychosis negatively affects the brain, so if a schizophrenic patient has been symptomatic for decades, his or her brain may have suffered so much damage that medications are not able to treat the condition. If medications are effective, patient often requires high doses for long periods of time. However, if a young, healthy patient comes to the hospital with a "first break," he or she is more likely to show a good response within days to relatively low doses of antipsychotics.

In 1954, a landmark study was published in Birmingham, England. They found similar results as the Swiss team: 25.9% of patients experienced a complete recovery, while 40.7% showed a partial recovery. In their discussion, they made a profound observation: ". . . in no case was the content of the psychosis changed. The schizophrenic and paraphrenic patients continued to be subject to delusions and hallucinations, though they appeared to be less disturbed by them." Essentially, the British psychiatrists replicated the effects in people that earlier scientists found in the rats that were conditioned to escape the electric shocks. Both groups were cognitively aware of an upsetting reality, but the antipsychotics made them less emotionally distressed.

Chlorpromazine gained popularity among psychiatrists in Canada before the United States. Most of these Canadian physicians had fled Nazi persecution in the 1930s and 1940s. A psychiatrist named Heinz Lehmann, working in Montreal, first experimented with the drug on a group of brave nursing students. They reported feeling more calm, but, did not show a decline in cognitive function. He published results involving the administration of high-dose chlorpromazine to psychotic patients. Over the course of several months, he noted a 66% positive response rate.

After Smith, Kline and French marketed chlorpromazine as Thorazine in 1954, the Food and Drug Administration (FDA) was reluctant to approve the drug for psychiatric uses. It was introduced in the United States for surgical purposes, mostly as an antiemetic to address nausea. There was also some initial reluctance among some American psychiatrists to shift toward a medical treatment to psychosis. The leading members of the psychiatric community at the time had studied directly under Sigmund Freud, the founder of psychoanalysis. They, therefore, leaned more toward psychoanalytic explanations of psychosis. They were interested in uncovering early childhood trauma to explain the psychotic behavior seen in adulthood. Therefore, the understanding and treatment of the illness were accomplished by psychoanalysis, which involved a patient lying on a couch, speaking spontaneously without direction, while the psychiatrist analyzed the patient's thoughts and tried to uncover the childhood trauma. It was difficult for them to accept that psychosis could be treated by taking a pill. It shifted the model of psychiatric illness from psychological to biological, like any other medical condition. Other psychiatrists conversely, particularly younger psychiatrists working in state hospitals, welcomed chlorpromazine as a solution to the overcrowded and at times dangerous condition of the facilities.

However, after several years, various interests in the United States pressured the psychiatric community to adopt chlorpromazine as a treatment for serious mental illnesses. Patients' families heard news from abroad about the benefits of the "wonder drug," and they were frustrated by the lack of success of traditional psychoanalytic practices. Psychoanalysis, after all, had serious problems. First of all, it was not effective for people with serious mental illnesses, like schizophrenia. It remained popular for decades and is still practiced today, but it is now used for patients with anxiety, depression, or personality disorders. Even Freud conceded that psychoanalysis did not cure schizophrenia. Another problem with psychoanalysis was that it was too labor-intensive. Each patient required about 40 minutes of a psychiatrist's time, roughly four times weekly. In the 1950s, there were over 550,000 patients in psychiatric hospitals in the Unites States. Clearly psychoanalysis was not an effective way to treat the country's mentally ill. As discussed earlier, many of these patients were administered treatments that most people would regard as inhumane, like insulin-shock therapy and prefrontal lobotomies. The "treatment" offered by the asylums prior to antipsychotic medications was essentially treatment for patients' families and society who were unable to care for the seriously mentally ill. State hospitals were overcrowded and often dangerous. Therefore, patient advocates were eager for patients to be treated with chlorpromazine.

At about the same time, in the early 1950s, another drug was analyzed for its potential in psychiatry. Reserpine was a medicine that had been used in Indian medicine for centuries. Derived from the plant *Rauwolfia serpentina*, it was given to patients with high fever, snake bites, insomnia, and psychosis. While reserpine was of most interest to the medical community for its antihypertensive properties, psychiatrists were curious about its potential for decreasing psychotic symptoms. Scientists were still decades from discovering the precise mechanism of action of either drug; it is now known that both drugs' psychiatric applications are due to the effects on the dopamine system. Whereas chlorpromazine blocks dopamine at the receptor in the brain, reserpine depletes the amount of dopamine in circulation.

Nathan Kline was a leader of American psychiatry at the time. He is best known for his contributions to psychoanalytic practice, but as the research director of Rockland State Hospital, a large state hospital, Kline began giving reserpine to hospitalized patients. He wrote a paper in 1954 that extolled the benefits of the drug, specifically in the decrease in assaults and aggressive behavior on the units. However, given that reserpine was being developed as a treatment for high blood pressure, it is not surprising that a side effect Kline found was the patients who took the drug experienced dangerously low blood pressures, leading to dizziness and fainting. As a result, reserpine never became a popular treatment because chlorpromazine achieved similar results with fewer side effects.

Pressure to reform the system also came from Smith, Kline and French, which stood to profit financially if Thorazine were accepted as a mainstream treatment. And profit they did. After several years of dragging their feet, by 1955, American psychiatrists began using Thorazine to treat major mental illnesses. Smith, Kline and French earned $75 million that year alone. American psychiatrists preferred to call the medications "tranquilizers" instead of "neuroleptics," which was the accepted term in Europe.

As a result of chlorpromazine's dissemination to thousands of patients, an enormous number were able to recover enough to be discharged from the hospital, beginning the era of "deinstitutionalization" discussed elsewhere. Between 1955 and 1965, 50 million patients were prescribed Thorazine. Over the first 20 years when antipsychotics were widely used, the number of patients in psychiatric hospitals decreased from 550,000 in 1955 to 200,000 in 1975.

It is also important to understand how the development of antipsychotics fit into the broader historical context of psychopharmacology. At about the same time when chlorpromazine was discovered, scientists began to use medications to treat patients with other mental illnesses. Lithium had been discussed as a treatment for mania since the late 19th century, but its potential was largely untapped. Researchers began testing it again in the 1940s and 1950s, and by the late 1960s, lithium was a commonly prescribed medication. It remains the first-line treatment for bipolar disorder. Antidepressants as well were being synthesized and researched in the 1950s. Benzodiazepines, including Valium and Xanax, now commonly used to treat anxiety, were developed in the 1960s. Antipsychotics were just one of a number of classes of medications that were driving the concept of mental illness into the general medical domain. For the first time, psychiatric patients were understood to have neurochemical disturbances that could be addressed with psychopharmacological solutions.

SIDE EFFECTS EMERGE

As early as 1952, however, patients and physicians began to understand that chlorpromazine, the new "miracle drug," as it was often called, had serious side effects. Movement disorders, also called extrapyramidal symptoms (EPS), described in detail elsewhere in this text, were informally discussed among psychiatrists. These included acute dystonia (sudden stiffness, often very painful), Parkinsonism (symptoms similar to patients with Parkinson's disease), and akathisia (the feeling of restlessness, very uncomfortable for patients).

In 1954, Swiss researcher Hans Steck and German psychiatrist Hans-Joachim Haase independently published the first formal descriptions of movement disorders. The early reports described a decreased ability to initiate movement, mask-like facial expression, and rigidity. Researchers concluded that when patients were given higher doses, they were more likely to develop these side effects.

An early term for antipsychotics, still used occasionally today, is "neuroleptics." "Neuro" refers to the central nervous system, and "leptic" is derived from the Greek, "to take hold." Antipsychotics were given this name because patients who suffered from EPS appeared as if something "took hold" of their nervous system. In the early days of antipsychotic administration, the development of EPS was thought to be a sign that the antipsychotic was working and at the correct dose. In 1955, a psychiatrist introduced the term "neuroleptic" and assigned it to all drugs in the same class. In the 1960s, however, the theory that the emergence of EPS implied clinical efficacy of the medication was debunked. Studies showed no relationship between when patients benefit from the psychiatric effects of antipsychotics and when they experience neurological side effects.

In the mid-1950s, the first reports of what would later be known as tardive dyskinesia (TD) were published in Europe. As discussed elsewhere, TD is a long-term EPS that involves involuntary movements like lip-smacking and rocking of the upper body. It is not painful, but it is generally very distressing and embarrassing for patients. Worse still, TD often does not resolve after an antipsychotic is discontinued.

Danish psychiatrists coined the term "tardive dyskinesia" in 1964. "Dyskinesia" referred to the abnormal movements described previously. "Tardive" was meant to convey the late-occurring nature of the side effect. It was noted early on that this unfortunate side effect could occur for up to two years after antipsychotics were stopped. The risks of developing TD are related to the dose and length of treatment. Therefore, the extent of TD was not fully known when it was first described in the 1950s and 1960s, because patients had only taken antipsychotics for no more than a decade. By now, enough patients have been on high doses of antipsychotics for many decades so that psychiatrists better appreciate the nature of TD. By the 1980s and 1990s, a large percentage of the state hospital patients, especially the elderly, had some degree of TD. After all, the patients who remained in the state hospitals during deinstitutionalization were the most treatment-resistant and therefore sickest patients. These are the patients that required the highest dose of antipsychotics and had received those high doses for decades. They were therefore most at risk for TD. Indeed, it was the concern about TD that drove the antipsychotic market in the direction of the newer, atypical antipsychotics, which are less likely to cause TD. Currently, many more atypical than typicals are prescribed. Psychiatrists are especially hesitant to prescribe typical antipsychotics to younger patients, because the theory is that they will need many years of treatment and therefore be at a higher risk of TD. However, as discussed elsewhere in this text, the newer atypical agents are more likely to cause metabolic side effects and diabetes. Diabetes is the leading cause of blindness, kidney failure, and limb amputations. Therefore, in the coming decades, as TD is replaced by these metabolic complications as the scourge of elderly patients in psychiatric hospitals, the pendulum may switch back to the older, typical agents.

The rare but life-threatening side effect, called neuroleptic malignant syndrome, which involved muscle rigidity, high temperatures, and delirium, was first described in the 1960s.

COMPETITION FOR CHLORPROMAZINE

In 1958, the company Haase and Janssen developed haloperidol with the trade name Haldol, which became the most commonly used antipsychotic and is still one of the most frequently prescribed antipsychotics used today. Paul Janssen, the lead researcher, synthesized haloperidol in an attempt to produce an opioid pain medication, but it was found to produce the type of movement disorders seen in the administration of high-dose chlorpromazine. Within months of its discovery, Janssen gave samples of haloperidol to Paul Divry and Jean Bobon, psychiatrists working at hospitals affiliated with the University of Liège in Belgium. The major advantage of haloperidol is that it is not as sedating as chlorpromazine. Patients were able to take full doses of the medication, obtain relief from their psychotic symptoms, but continued to function throughout the day. Chlorpromazine is a very sedating drug, so patients who required significant doses were often too tired to fully recover their pre-illness level of activity. However, the disadvantage of haloperidol, noticed immediately by the researchers and the first psychiatrists to use the drug, was the pronounced movement side effects. EPS were the expectation, not the unwelcome side effect.

Janssen proudly described one of the first patients given haloperidol by Divry and Bobon. He was a student and the son of a physician in practice near the hospital. He was admitted due to paranoia and agitation, common reasons young men with schizophrenia are admitted to psychiatric hospitals early in their illness. He was given a 10-mg injection of haloperidol to rapidly address his symptoms, which Janssen said dramatically improved his condition. He then took a 1-mg pill every day for the next seven years and was able to carry on with his studies, get married, and had children. He then stopped taking haloperidol and was readmitted to the hospital three weeks later.

Chemists then began to search for an antipsychotic that did not cause EPS. Clozapine was first synthesized in 1958 and was the first of what are now called the second-generation antipsychotics or atypical antipsychotics. Clinical trials in Europe confirmed that the drug maintained antipsychotic properties but was not as frequently associated with EPS, which was a remarkable finding. Further, clozapine was found in some studies to actually work better than other previously manufactured antipsychotics in that it reduced symptoms of psychosis in patients that did not respond to other medications. However, shortly after clozapine began to be widely used, a troubling finding was reported in Finland.

In 1975, an article in the medical journal *Lancet* described 18 patients who were prescribed clozapine and developed agranulocytosis, a depletion of neutrophils, a type of white blood cells. White blood cells are responsible for fighting infections, and neutrophils specifically target bacteria. Therefore, patients who suffer from agranulocytosis cannot effectively fight bacterial illness and are vulnerable to life-threatening infections. Nine of these 18 patients died.

This development led clozapine to be taken off the market in Finland and several other European countries. Research on the drug was also suspended.

However, interest in the drug resumed after TD grew to epidemic proportions in the 1980s. Clozapine was viewed as a potential solution to addressing psychosis without leading to TD, but the rare side effect involving white blood cells gave pause to psychiatrists. More research showed that clozapine was safe to give as long as patients' white blood cell count, and specifically their neutrophil count, is carefully monitored. Clozapine was approved by the FDA for use in the United States under the trade name Clozaril in 1988.

Clozapine had an additional effect that distinguished it from the typical antipsychotics. Clozapine was effective in treating the negative symptoms of schizophrenia in addition to the positive symptoms. As discussed elsewhere, positive symptoms are components of the illness that are present, whereas in non-affected individuals, they are not seen. These include hallucinations and delusions. Negative symptoms are elements of behaviors that are *not* seen in schizophrenia patients and that are present in non-affected individuals, including normal amount of motivation, normal speech, organized behavior, and appropriate socialization. Patients prescribed clozapine were noted not just to have decreased hallucinations and delusions but also to have more organized behavior and speech and better motivation and were able to maintain more normal relationships. The ability to target negative symptoms in addition to positive symptoms was found to a certain extent in all the second-generation or atypical antipsychotics. Scientists learned later that the biochemical reason for this advantage is that atypical antipsychotics operate on the serotonin system as well as the dopamine system, whereas typical antipsychotics work only on the dopamine system.

Clozapine, in addition to serving as the prototypic second-generation antipsychotic, emerged as an especially important medication for other reasons. Both initially and over time, clozapine was shown to reduce symptoms in patients who were treatment-resistant and did not respond to other medications. It is therefore considered more effective than any other antipsychotic, including the many antipsychotics that were developed decades after clozapine. This was demonstrated in the landmark Clinical Antipsychotic Trials of Clinical Effectiveness (CATIE) study that released its first findings in 2005. This was the largest and remains the most reliable study that compared the efficacy of the different antipsychotics. In addition to providing relief to patients who did not benefit from other antipsychotics, clozapine has also been shown to be the only antipsychotic to reduce the incidence of suicide.

In 1969, an important innovation in the delivery of antipsychotics was first made available for the U.S. consumers. Fluphenazine, under the trade name

Modecate, was distributed in a long-acting formulation. Prior to this, patients received medication in the form of pills or fast-acting injection. Due to the nature of the illnesses that antipsychotics treat, it is difficult for patients to take medications every day and even several times daily. If patients are acutely dangerous to themselves or others and refuse medications, they are given injections, but to receive long-term care in that manner is difficult, mostly because being held down and given a painful injection routinely are physically and emotionally traumatic for the patients. However, in 1969, the option to take one injection monthly and have a steady amount of medication in circulation appealed to many physicians and patients. The medication is essentially packaged in lipids that do not readily dissolve into the bloodstream. Instead, there is a slow release of the drug into the body that takes up to one month. Depot injections became a preferred method to administer antipsychotics to patients who were found by doctors or judges to be incapable of making rationale medical decisions and were therefore given antipsychotics over their objection. However, many patients who voluntarily accepted antipsychotics preferred long-acting depot injection, so they did not have to be bothered with taking pills regularly or risking a relapse if they were unable to access their prescriptions. Several antipsychotics later were made available in this formulation, including haloperidol, risperidone, olanzapine, and aripiprazole.

After clozapine, many other atypical antipsychotics were developed. They essentially have the same mechanisms of actions, but their side effect profiles differ slightly. Janssen was specifically interested in finding a drug that simultaneously blocks dopamine and serotonin. The hypothesis was that if both neurotransmitters were blocked, positive and negative symptoms of schizophrenia could be addressed with one agent that also caused less EPS. Risperidone was first synthesized in 1983 and approved by the FDA in 1994. Olanzapine was approved in 1996, and quetiapine was approved in 1997. Since then, over 10 atypical antipsychotics have reached the U.S. market.

Importantly, it was through antipsychotics that scientists were able to make important conclusions about the biological basis of mental illnesses. Through painstaking work, antipsychotics were shown to block the dopamine receptor in the brain. This led therefore to the "dopamine hypothesis," formally put forth by researchers at Johns Hopkins University in 1974, although it had already been discussed in psychiatric circles for several years before then. Essentially, they postulated that if antipsychotics block dopamine and if antipsychotics treat psychosis, then psychosis must be caused by excessive dopamine activity. Further supporting the link between dopamine and schizophrenia, they noted that drugs like amphetamines, which increase levels of dopamine, triggered psychosis in certain individuals. This idea dominated academic psychiatry for over 30 years, until other hypotheses were introduced that suggested more complicated explanations of psychosis, involving other receptors in the brain. Starting in the 1990s, glutamate, a neurotransmitter that binds to the N-methyl-D-aspartate (NMDA) receptor found throughout the body, has been postulated to be equally relevant, or even more so, to the biological basis of schizophrenia than dopamine. At the center of this theory is the fact that certain drugs, such as phencyclidine (PCP), which affect the NMDA system, produce a state similar to acutely symptomatic schizophrenia, including positive and negative symptoms of the disease.

Our knowledge and understanding of how antipsychotics work have evolved significantly since their inception in the 1950s. In the 1990s, innovations in the field of biotechnology have allowed researchers to label chemicals radioactively. This makes it possible to trace the movements of the drugs in the brain and analyze specific chemical properties at respective receptors. Through these techniques, researchers discovered that there are different types of dopamine receptors, and different antipsychotics behave differently. The Dopamine-2 (D2) receptor was shown to be the most relevant dopamine subtype receptor in the brain, as antipsychotics bind to this receptor preferentially. Some antipsychotics, called "high-potency" antipsychotics, were shown to occupy a higher proportion of the brain's D2 receptors, whereas "low potency" antipsychotics, like chlorpromazine or clozapine, occupy as smaller percentage. Scientists then tied this discovery with the drugs' observed side effect profile; the antipsychotics with higher dopamine occupancy rates (blocking a larger percentage of receptors) are more likely to cause EPS or Parkinsonism. This is logical because Parkinson's disease is caused by the degeneration of dopamine cells in a specific part of the brain called the substantia nigra.

HOW ANTIPSYCHOTICS ARE USED TODAY: BRIDGING PAST AND FUTURE

In the United States today, patients are prescribed antipsychotics in a variety of settings. Due to deinstitutionalization, the majority of patients who are prescribed antipsychotics are in the community. Many patients are treated with antipsychotics in emergency rooms and acute psychiatric units in general medical hospitals, and some remain in long-term state hospitals. As discussed elsewhere, many patients are prescribed antipsychotics in jails and prisons.

The conditions of state hospitals have improved significantly over the past 60 years, when the realities of the patients' experiences were brought to the attention of the American public. The principal reason for the improvement has been a greater respect for the rights and civil liberties of the mentally ill, borne out of the increased attention to civil rights for other disenfranchised citizens that dominated in the 1960s and 1970s. This trend has taken the form both of gradual improvement and of swift changes brought on by judicial action. In the case *Wyatt v. Stickney* (1972), a judge in Alabama determined that patients in state hospitals had the right to a certain standard of care. This involved proper staff and set a minimum of two psychiatrists and 12 nurses for every 250 patients. This may not seem like a very favorable benchmark for patients, and today this would translate to a very poorly staffed facility, but prior to this ruling, some state hospitals were woefully underfunded and provided care much below the level set by the standard. At times, psychiatrists were responsible for thousands of patients, and there was not extensive therapeutic programming in place. This meant that patients were not given individual attention, and their recovery was limited. Today, patients at state hospitals are consistently followed by psychiatrists and have extensive therapeutic activities and groups.

The majority of patients with serious mental illnesses that are prescribed antipsychotics live in the community. They live in private residences or various types of supportive housing, which is housing that is designed for clients with serious mental illnesses. This housing is generally paid for with patient's public benefits, like Supplemental Security Income (SSI) or Social Security Disability (SSD). They usually provide counselors on the premises who can support patients, assist with everyday problems, and respond quickly to crises. Unfortunately, many patients with mental illnesses, especially in urban centers, are homeless. This includes the populations in homeless shelters or street homeless individuals.

As discussed elsewhere in the text, a primary problem faced by psychiatrists who prescribe antipsychotics today is patients who are frequently noncompliant with treatment. Many people consistently cycle between shelters, emergency rooms, and inpatient units, as their symptoms worsen due to medication noncompliance and, frequently, substance use. They often are not in the community consistently enough to maintain relationships with mental health providers. An additional problem with the population is they do not live anywhere long enough to apply for and receive consistent benefits, like SSI or SSD, to allow admission to appropriate supportive housing. This pattern of care—treatment exclusively in acute settings during periods of decompensation—is extremely costly for society because it involves significant health resources, but, more importantly, it is bad for the patient. Frequent psychotic episodes lead to a worse prognosis, as discussed elsewhere in this text. Therefore, a major task of today's psychiatrists is educating and encouraging patients to take better control of their mental illnesses. This can be helped by long-acting depot antipsychotics and the use of clozapine, which has been shown to be the most effective antipsychotic.

Over the past decade, public officials have fully appreciated the problem that treating mental illness poses to the correctional systems. As discussed elsewhere, 15–20% of the incarcerated population has a serious mental illness, which does not include personality disorders, substance use disorders, or most depressive and anxiety disorders. Antipsychotics are widely used in correctional settings, requiring jails and prisons to employ large numbers of mental health professionals. It is clear that this approach is not ideal. Patients with serious mental illnesses do worse in correctional settings, and the correctional systems do not specialize in mental health administration. Therefore, there has been significant momentum across the political spectrum to reduce the number of mentally ill prisoners. This involves the diversion of mentally ill offenders from the justice system to the mental health system, at various points along the road to incarceration. Police are being trained to identify mental illnesses and bring patients to the hospital instead of to the police station, especially when they are found committing "quality of life" crimes like public urination and loitering. Furthermore, many municipalities have established specialized mental health courts, with judges who have training in mental health. Through these courts, after people have been booked and charged with a crime, they are diverted to mandated treatment in hospitals or in the community. This way, the treatment of mental illnesses and administration of antipsychotics can take place in facilities designed for that purpose, instead of prisons that are designed to secure dangerous criminals.

Another trend in the treatment of serious mental illnesses is the improvement of mental health awareness of municipal employees who work with the homeless populations. A greater effort is being made nationwide to identify mental illness and facilitate treatment, when the mental illness itself is preventing the patient from secure consistent housing. This involves the homeless population in shelters and the street homeless population. For various reasons, either due to the paranoid delusions of the mentally ill homeless individual or the dangerous nature of shelters, many homeless people avoid shelters at all costs. As a result, each year, several homeless people, many with serious mental illness, freeze to death in the winter. This is a deplorable reality in a country with ample ability to provide warm and safe facilities for everyone during inclement weather. In January 2016, Governor Andrew Cuomo of New York highlighted this issue by issuing an executive order that empowered law enforcement to use, in part, mental health law to remove homeless individuals from the street in temperatures below 32 degrees F.

As described earlier, the treatment of serious mental illnesses has a long history. It has involved spiritual remedies, punitive measures, and primitive treatments based on faulty hypotheses that led to far more damage than recovery. Antipsychotic medications have dominated the treatment of serious mental illnesses for the past 60 years. They have facilitated significant progress and, most notably, allowed treatment to transition from the locked doors of state asylums to the outpatient doctor's office. Antipsychotic medications cause much less damage than earlier forms of treatment, including insulin-shock treatment and lobotomies; however, the side effects are real, and must be taken seriously by psychiatrists and patients. It has become abundantly clear in the recent decades that the most effective antipsychotic—defined as a treatment of psychotic illness—is actually a robust medical and social response. This involves not only antipsychotic medications but also tools that help patients remain compliant in the community, a network of outreach workers that identify and engage mentally ill in the community and a justice system that diverts the mentally ill from corrections to mental health treatment as much as possible.

Chapter 4

How Antipsychotics Work

Thus far we have taken a general look at antipsychotics as a whole and a few individual medications and explored the history of their development. Their ability to act in the body and make changes in psychotic symptoms has been touched on but needs to be examined deeper. This can seem like an overwhelming task, as antipsychotics work in a multitude of ways, and not all of their mechanisms are clearly understood. Not to mention, the body and its ability to function and regulate itself as a whole, in a normal state, is quite an amazing feat. But its ability to adjust, regulate, and adapt to environmental factors and medications is remarkable and can be understood on different levels of difficulty. The antipsychotics have been developed and have evolved in response to the evolution of the hypotheses about psychotic disorders and the neurotransmitters that may be involved in causing them. In order to understand how these medications may actually be efficacious, it is important to have an understanding of the neurotransmitters and what their biological role is as well as the pathways that they act in. Then one can understand where in that pathway the antipsychotics target and modulate the neurotransmitters, which has an effect on symptoms.

Prior to that, even more basic than understanding how the neurotransmitters act in the brain, one must have some baseline understanding of the various roles of different parts of the brain. This chapter will explore how antipsychotics work in the body on a chemical basis in order to give a better groundwork for understanding how they interact with the body, causing improvements and unwanted side effects.

PARTS OF THE BRAIN

To begin understanding how antipsychotics work in the body, it is important to lay the groundwork first and have some sort of understanding of the parts of the brain and how they operate. Antipsychotics' main mechanism of action takes place in the brain. The medications target different parts of the brain to cause effect on some of the psychotic symptoms that have been mentioned in earlier chapters. The brain is a quite complex organ, thought to be the control center of the body. Here the goal will be to gain a simplified understanding of some of the major roles of various parts of the brain in order to understand where and how antipsychotics may work.

The brain is part of the central nervous system. The fact that there is a central nervous system suggests that there are other nervous systems as well, which there are. They are all interconnected, and since psychiatric diseases and their treatment can have an impact on the central, peripheral, and autonomic nervous systems, it is best to lay the groundwork for all before discussing the brain itself. In simplified terms, the nervous system as a whole is the part of an animal's (in this case, human's) body that is responsible for coordinating all involuntary and voluntary actions. It does this by transmitting signals to and from different parts of the body. The nervous system is subdivided into a central nervous system and peripheral nervous system. The central nervous system is made up of the brain and the spinal cord. It can be thought of as mostly receiving information from the peripheral nervous system and various parts of the body that it processes and coordinates in order to respond with a voluntary action. The peripheral nervous system is basically the rest of the nerves, including all the nerves and ganglia (a cluster of nerve cells), that exist outside of the brain and spinal cord. Its main function is to connect the brain and spinal cord to the rest of the body and to serve as the route through which information is transmitted from the periphery to the center of control, the brain and spinal cord. It has some nerves that carry information to the central nervous system and others that carry information away from the central nervous system.

The brain can be grossly thought of as being divided into four lobes—frontal, parietal, occipital, and temporal. This classification was originally thought to be based solely on anatomical location but over the years has been shown to be related to different brain functions. The brain is also divided into hemispheres or halves. So there is a right side of the brain and a left side of the brain. Each side of the brain has one of each lobe, so on the right side of the brain there is a frontal, parietal, temporal, and occipital lobe, and the same for the left. There could be, and have been, entire books written to describe the various lobes of the brain and their different roles in functionality, and many of them are still being studied. For the purposes of this book, it is only necessary to have a broader and briefer understanding of the more generalized roles of the different lobes. In order to grasp an understanding of how antipsychotics have an impact on different brain structures and pathways, leading to changes in behavior, it is important to have a basic understanding of the roles of some key parts of the brain that are involved in the pathology.

The frontal lobes are, as the name would suggest, located at the front of the brain, one in the right hemisphere and one in the left hemisphere. They play a key role in conscious thought and executive functioning. Executive functioning refers to the ability to manage cognitive process, to problem solve, plan, and put into action. Damage to the frontal lobes often results in mood changes and lack of inhibition, leading to socially inappropriate behavior. In medicine, the story of Phineas Gage is often used to help impart this information on learners. The actual facts of his story have probably been twisted and misconstrued over the years; however, it is still a helpful teaching tool and has become part of medical folklore. The story is that Phineas Gage was an American railroad construction foreman in the 1840s, who met a railroad accident. He had a large iron rod driven through his head, destroying a lot of his left frontal lobe. It was said, by family and friends, that his personality drastically changed after the accident and that he went from a polite, hardworking man to a lazy and rude person for the rest of his life. The frontal lobes also contain the majority of dopamine-sensitive neurons in the cerebral cortex, which is the outer layer of the brain. The role of dopamine in psychosis and with antipsychotics will be discussed in detail later in the chapter, but just knowing that there are a large number of dopamine neurons in the frontal lobes means that the frontal lobes will be crucial to psychosis and its treatment.

The parietal lobes play a major role in integrating sensory information that is received from various sources, including the processing of taste, temperature, and touch. While this lobe is not responsible for the sense of sight it does process some of that information and plays a large role in visuospatial processing. Parts of the parietal lobe also have a major role in language processing. Damage in the parietal lobes could lead to mistakes in processing visual and spatial information.

The occipital lobe is located in the back and is the lobe that is responsible for the sense of sight. Its functionality is subdivided into different areas of the lobe, so damage to different parts of the lobe will cause various types of either alterations or loss of sight.

Finally, the temporal lobe plays a large role in smell and sound. Similar to the occipital lobe, it is responsible for processing and integrating this information, so damage to specific areas of the lobe will cause different alterations in smell and sound. It is also responsible for processing more complex stimuli such as facial recognition, language recognition, and comprehension and the encoding of more long-term memories and the emotions that are associated with them. This lobe has many different functions, and, therefore, damage here can produce different symptoms depending on the portion of the lobe that is affected.

This is a simplified understanding of the different lobes of the brain and various functions of the brain, and as you focus on more specific areas of the brain, the functions also become more specific. However, this should give a good baseline understanding that can be called upon when thinking about the various neurotransmitters that play a role in psychiatric illnesses and antipsychotic medications to help better understand their effects.

WHAT ARE NEUROTRANSMITTERS AND WHAT DO THEY DO?

The body operates in order to attempt to always be in a state of balance, called homeostasis. There are multiple systems in place within the body that are regulated so that internal conditions remain stable and relatively constant. As is well known, the brain is somewhat of the master controller. It receives signals from various parts of the body, interprets them, and then sends out signals to perform an action. The brain communicates with itself and the rest of the body through the nervous system, using neurons as the messengers, to send signals. Neurotransmitters are naturally occurring chemicals that are produced within the body and serve to transmit the signals that the neurons send to each other. Neurons are not physically connected to one another; they are joined by synapses and are separated by a synaptic cleft. Neurotransmitters are sent from one neuron to another via synaptic vesicles through the synaptic cleft. There are receptors on the receiving neuron that accept specific neurotransmitters. So, for instance, when dopamine is transmitted from one neuron to another, it is released from the first neuron in a synaptic vesicle. It then travels across the synaptic cleft and is received in a dopamine specific receptor on the next neuron. It cannot attach to a serotonin receptor or any other neurotransmitter receptor; it must be a dopamine receptor. Once attached to a receptor, neurotransmitters generally have either an inhibitory or excitatory effect on the receiving neuron. This means that once the neurotransmitter is received, a message is understood or unlocked, and the response will be either an increase in the receiving neuron's function or a decrease in the neuron's function.

There are more than 100 neurotransmitters that have been identified and likely many more out there. They play a large role in nearly every day-to-day function that the body performs and are essential to maintain that normal functioning. There is a general flow and transmission of neurotransmitters that helps to maintain the homeostasis that the body is constantly working toward maintaining. However, when something pathological occurs, it can include either an increase or decrease in neurotransmitters, which would lead to an alteration of functioning. There are many disorders and diseases that involve either an increase or decrease in one or more neurotransmitters, so many of the medications we use regularly work by altering neurotransmitter activity. Psychiatric disorders are no different, and many of them, including psychotic disorders, are hypothesized to have some type of alteration in neurotransmitters, so the medications, including antipsychotics, target specific neurotransmitters. Those neurotransmitters and their normal role and hypothesized role in disease and impact by antipsychotics will be discussed in the following pages.

NEUROTRANSMITTERS AFFECTED BY ANTIPSYCHOTICS

Two of the most important neurotransmitters in psychiatric disorders that have become targets of treatment are dopamine and serotonin. However, there are many other neurotransmitters that are also impacted by medications used to treat psychiatric disorders, including antipsychotics. The following pages will explore in detail dopamine and serotonin as important neurotransmitters in psychiatric disorders and as modifiable by antipsychotics. They will also explore some other, currently less prominent but perhaps with much potential, neurotransmitters that are hypothesized to be involved in psychiatric disorders and are affected by some antipsychotics.

Dopamine

Dopamine is a neurotransmitter involved in multiple different brain systems. Dopamine also has many vital roles outside of the central nervous system, but for the purposes of this book, the focus will be on its many roles in the brain. In order to have a greater understanding of how dopamine works in the central nervous system and the periphery, it is important to understand how the neurotransmitter is produced and regulated. Dopamine synthesis begins with the amino acid tyrosine. It is transported in dopamine neurons and then becomes hydroxylated to form L-dopa. Hydroxylation refers to a biochemical process of adding a hydroxyl group (an oxygen and hydrogen) to an organic compound. This hydroxylation allows the tyrosine to transform into a functionally different compound. Because this step changes the function of the compound, it is considered the rate-limiting step in the production of dopamine. The rate-limiting step in the production of different compounds plays an important role in controlling how much of the compound is available for use in the body. For dopamine, the hydroxylation from tyrosine to L-dopa is the key point of regulation for the eventual availability of dopamine in the body. This rate-limiting step is essential for the production of dopamine to be able to respond to alterations in storage, release, metabolism, or impulse flow that is induced by functional demands or drugs. This is how the body can alter its own production of the neurotransmitter, by hydroxylating more tyrosine, in order to regulate its level of dopamine and attempt to maintain homeostasis. L-dopa undergoes another step before becoming dopamine in the periphery; however, peripheral L-dopa can cross the blood-brain barrier and then rapidly decarboxylate to dopamine. Decarboxylation is a biochemical process that removes a carboxyl group, which is one carbon, two oxygen, and one hydrogen (COOH), and releases carbon dioxide. Once dopamine is produced and has been transported to a dopamine neuron, it can be stored within a synaptic vesicle in the dopamine neuron. In the dopamine neuron and within a synaptic vesicle, it can be metabolized by monoamine oxidase. It also could be metabolized outside of the neuron by catechol-O-methyltransferase. Dopamine can be broken down by either of these two chemical compounds. As mentioned earlier, the body is always trying to maintain some type of homeostasis, some type of balance. Part of the way that this is maintained is by the regulation and control that the various systems in the body attempt to enact. Similarly, the dopamine neuron is part of one of those systems; it is a dynamic unit that is constantly working to try to maintain homeostasis, including a stable level of dopamine, and it utilizes these biochemical processes to control the amount of dopamine created and metabolized in an attempt to maintain that homeostasis. It is hypothesized that at least one of the factors playing a role in the presentation of schizophrenia is an imbalance of dopamine, showing how important that regulation and homeostasis can be to daily functioning. It is still not completely understood why changes in dopamine would cause all of the psychotic symptoms of psychosis, but understanding dopamine's role in the body helps to frame this hypothesis.

Pathways and Functions

Dopamine plays an important role in facilitating many different functions in the body. Some of these roles include motor control, reward, motivation, cognitive control, arousal, and lactation. Dopamine's interactions through its various tracts in the brain facilitate motor behavior. These behaviors promoted by dopamine are based on seeking and finding rewards; they are driven to seek out food and other rewarding activities. Dopamine has been shown to clearly be associated with the pleasure and reward system and is part of our understanding of addiction. Many addictive drugs like cocaine, amphetamines, ecstasy, and other psychostimulants have been shown to have their effect by increasing dopamine in the brain, leading to more pleasure, reward, and eventual addiction in some cases. Dopamine has a few small and specific areas in the brain where the cell bodies are located, but it has projections and pathways that reach to many different areas of the brain. The role of dopamine can be generally categorized based on where the cell bodies lie. There are four basic dopaminergic pathways to understand in order to grasp the function of dopamine in the brain. They are the mesolimbic pathway, mesocortical pathway, nigrostriatal pathway, and tuberoinfundibular pathway. Each pathway has a different function, and, therefore, their role in psychotic disorders and how they are impacted by antipsychotics vary for each path. First, it is important to understand how they work in the healthy individual and then we will look at how they might be impacted by a psychotic disorder and where antipsychotics would target different pathways for treatment.

The ventral tegmental area is an area of the brain located in the midbrain that plays a large role as a pleasure center. It has multiple different neuronal pathways that stem from it, and one of its major neurotransmitters is dopamine. It houses many dopamine neuron cells that project to various areas in the brain. Specifically it has two major dopamine pathways, called the mesolimbic pathway and the mesocortical pathway, both of which are thought to be altered in schizophrenia. The mesolimbic pathway is a connection from the ventral tegmental area to the nucleus accumbens. This pathway is also sometimes referred to as the reward pathway, and it seems to be the most significant neural pathway involved in reward and addiction. The mesocortical pathway is a dopaminergic pathway that connects the ventral tegmentum to the cerebral cortex. The cerebral cortex is the outer layer of brain tissue, also referred to as gray matter, that covers the entire brain. It has many roles that impact human behavior, interactions, and individual and external awareness. Some of its key roles include memory, attention, awareness, thought, language, and consciousness. The different roles of the cortex vary depending on where (which lobe) they are located. The mesocortical pathway connects to the cerebral cortex, particularly in the frontal lobes. This pathway is essential to a specific part of the frontal lobe, the dorsolateral prefrontal cortex, and is involved in cognitive control, motivation, and emotional response.

The other dopamine pathways in the brain that are thought to be either altered in schizophrenia or impacted by antipsychotics are not located in the ventral tegmentum. The tuberoinfundibular pathway refers to a connection from a group of dopamine neurons in the arcuate nucleus, located in the hypothalamus, that connects to the pituitary gland. This is a major endocrine gland located at the base of the brain that secretes multiple hormones that are involved in growth, blood pressure, metabolism, and some aspects of pregnancy and nursing, among others. This pathway marks one of dopamine's more unique roles but is still connected to psychosis and its treatment. In this pathway dopamine serves to regulate the secretion of prolactin, which is a hormone with many different roles, well known for its role in lactation. Dopamine functions as an inhibitor to prolactin secretion; so if there is a decrease in dopamine, there can be an increase in blood prolactin levels.

The final dopamine pathway that is thought to play a role in psychotic disorders or their treatment is the nigrostriatal pathway. This pathway is a dopaminergic pathway that connects the substantia nigra with the dorsal striatum. The substantia nigra is located deep in the brain, in the midbrain, and plays a role in reward, addiction, and movement. The dorsal striatum serves as the primary input to the basal ganglia, which is heavily involved in the control of voluntary movements. This pathway from the substantia nigra to the dorsal striatum is particularly involved in the basal ganglia motor loop and plays a large role in the production and control of voluntary movements. One of the most common neurodegenerative disorders, second only to Alzheimer's disease, is Parkinson's disease, where the main pathology is found in this basal ganglia motor loop. In Parkinson's disease, there is a loss of dopamine neurons in the substantia nigra that leads to a decrease of dopamine in this basal ganglia motor loop and causes many of the motor symptoms of Parkinson's disease.

This provides a basic understanding of the four major dopaminergic pathways in the brain that are either hypothesized to be altered in psychotic disorders or will be altered by the use of antipsychotic medications. So, there are four different dopamine pathways in the brain that are located in different areas and have different functions. Within those different pathways, dopamine is transported and then accepted by a dopamine receptor, but not all dopamine receptors are created equal; they are divided into different classes. There are five types of dopamine receptors, but they are divided into two major classes: D1 and D2 receptors. The distinction is based on biochemical observations showing that one type of dopamine receptor is able to modulate a certain chemical (adenylyl cyclase) and the other type is not. Later it has been discovered that there are multiple subtypes based on the structural, pharmacological, and biochemical properties of the receptors. They are now classified as D1 class, which includes D1 and D5 receptors, and D2 class, which includes D2, D3, and D4 receptors. This is mostly pertinent to this discussion because medications can and do target the specific receptor as opposed to all dopamine receptors. Understanding the details of how and why the receptors vary from each other is complicated and more appropriate for a biochemistry course. For the purposes of this book, it is important to understand where these different types of receptors might be located mostly. In general, dopamine receptors have broad expression in the brain and in the peripheral body. In the brain, D1 receptors are expressed in high density in the nigrostriatal, mesolimbic, and mesocortical areas, which include many of the areas that the four pathways previously mentioned traveled, except for the tuberoinfundibular. The D5 receptors are expressed in relatively low levels in many brain regions. D2 receptors are found in significant levels in the striatum, nucleus accumbens, olfactory tubercle, substantia nigra, ventral tegmental area, and hypothalamus, among others. The D3 and D4 receptors have more limited patterns of expression in the brain. Clearly there will be a high density of D1 and D2 receptors in nearly all of the pathways thought to be involved in psychotic disorders, with a smaller expression of D3, D4, and D5 receptors. This baseline information about dopamine, its pathways, and receptors gives a basic understanding of how dopamine operates in the healthy, functioning body. Dopamine is hypothesized to be altered in schizophrenia and other psychiatric disorders, so having a good understanding of how it is naturally transported and regulated throughout the body is crucial to understanding what happens when it is not working right. Next we will look at how dopamine and its pathways may be altered in psychiatric disorders, particularly in schizophrenia.

How Psychiatric Disorders Affect Dopamine

Once you understand how neurotransmitters operate and some of the functions that they help regulate, like cognition, thought process, emotions, reward, and executive functioning, it is not a stretch to imagine that if there is either too much or too little of some of them, it could be linked with psychiatric disorders. While it is thought that many psychiatric disorders are caused by an alteration of neurotransmitters, still the molecular mechanisms underlying the disorders are often not completely understood. However, there are many, regularly evolving hypotheses about them that generally involve some type of neurotransmitter. And in order to understand the reasoning behind antipsychotics' mechanism of action and how they are thought to cause effects, one must understand what is thought to be the neurotransmitter abnormality that is being targeted. As mentioned previously, this can be difficult at times as the cause and abnormality in all psychotic disorders are not clearly understood. This is compounded by the fact that the detailed mechanism of action of all antipsychotics is not completely understood. In order to try to simplify this, it is easiest to examine what are thought to be the neurotransmitter abnormalities in schizophrenia and how the antipsychotics are thought to work in schizophrenia. This explanation can then be extrapolated to apply to other psychotic disorders. Further on in the book will be a more in-depth look at the specific uses of antipsychotics and their typical effects in certain disorders.

The oldest hypothesis about the origin of schizophrenia is a dopamine hypothesis. This evolved from clinical observations and was somewhat validated by using treatment with antipsychotics that altered dopamine in the brain. While this hypothesis does not attempt to explain the complexity of the disorder, it offers a direct relationship between the symptoms (psychosis) and the treatment (antipsychotics that alter dopamine). This hypothesis has evolved over the years and in more recent years has been challenged by other hypotheses. The original hypothesis was that schizophrenia was caused by hyperactivity of dopamine in the brain. This was largely based on the idea that psychostimulants that brought about psychotic symptoms activated dopamine receptors and that dopamine played an important role in the extrapyramidal movement system. Further supporting this dopamine hypothesis, it was suggested that stress played some role in the expression of schizophrenia. It is not that stress may lead to schizophrenia but was suggested that in individuals who are predisposed to schizophrenia, acute stress may cause an increase in dopamine that then leads to expression of the psychotic symptoms. To further support that, it seems that dopamine turnover in some parts of the brain is in fact greatly accelerated with stress. Thus far we have discussed the hypothesis that schizophrenia is caused by an overactivation of dopamine in the brain. However, as may be expected, it is more complex than just too much dopamine in the brain. If that were the case, then one would expect the typical antipsychotics, which are dopamine blockers, to cure all of the symptoms suffered with schizophrenia, which is not the case. Instead, the hypothesis has continued to evolve to suggest that there is a hyperactivity of dopamine in certain pathways of the brain and a decrease in activity of dopamine in other pathways of the brain.

The symptoms and presentation of schizophrenia were touched on earlier in the book, but the presentation is complex, and there is a variety of constellations of symptoms that can be seen. The two broad categories of symptoms are positive and negative symptoms. Recall from an earlier chapter that the positive symptoms refer to distortions in an individual's way of thinking, speaking, and perceiving their surroundings. The three large categories of positive symptoms include delusions, perceptual disturbances, and thought disorders. The negative symptoms refer to alterations in how an individual shows emotion and their cognition. Specifically, they refer to an inability to express their emotions, slowed cognition, and a decrease or lack of motivation. The dopaminergic pathways that were presented earlier in this chapter are thought to have different alterations in schizophrenia, some with an increase in dopamine and others with a decrease in dopamine, which would lead to both positive and negative symptoms.

The dopamine hypothesis of schizophrenia suggests that there is an excess of dopamine in the subcortical areas of the brain, meaning that there is a hyper-stimulation of D2 receptors in subcortical areas. It is thought that there is an overactivity of dopamine in the mesolimbic tract that is largely responsible for the positive symptoms of schizophrenia. In support of this hypothesis, there are studies looking at symptoms when there are either lesions or over-stimulation of the limbic system. It is suggested that impairment of the ability to filter out multiple stimuli and disturbances in behavior and affect may be the result of lesions in the limbic system. For instance, electrical stimulation of the dorsal hippocampus, which is part of the outflow of the limbic system, has been reported to produce positive symptoms of psychosis, including thought disorders and hallucinations. Other changes that have been seen with either stimulation or ablation in the limbic system are consistent with psychotic symptoms, including paranoia, depersonalization, perceptual dis-turbances, catatonia, and disturbances of mood and emotion. While these symptoms are not necessarily specific, combined with other information they help to support the hypothesis that positive psychotic symptoms are caused by an increase in dopamine in the mesolimbic tract. Contrasting with that overactivity in the mesolimbic tract, it is hypothesized that there is decreased activity of dopamine in the mesocortical tract. However, this hypothesis has further developed and changed over time, as research has advanced and people have observed the effects of antipsychotics. These observations have led to changes in the antipsychotics to attempt to make them more therapeutic. In the following pages we will examine first the typical antipsychotics and then the atypical antipsychotics and how they are thought to take effect and make changes to dopamine levels and cause effect in the human body, specifically in the brain.

How Typical Antipsychotics Affect Dopamine

There are two main ways that medications alter neurotransmitter activity. Some medications are considered agonists. This means that the medication can bind to a specific neurotransmitter receptor and cause the same reaction that the naturally produced neurotransmitter would. It will lead to an overall increase in the neurotransmitter and its effects. Other medications are consid-ered antagonists and have the opposite effect on the neurotransmitter. A medi-cation that is an antagonist binds to a specific neurotransmitter receptor but simply blocks the receptor instead of causing a biological response. When a medication works as an antagonist, it will lead to an overall decrease in the neurotransmitter and its effects on the body.

The typical antipsychotics have always been thought of in a rather simplified manner. They all share the quality of being dopamine antagonists, which is how they are hypothesized to take effect on psychotic disorders. Specifically, they block the D2 receptors in various parts of the brain. Many medications used to treat psychiatric illnesses and nearly all of the antipsychotics have more than one impact on the body. The typical antipsychotics all share the same main therapeutic goal, which is to block D2 receptors. However, all of the typical antipsychotics also have effects on some other receptors, and they are limited in how specific they can be with their dopamine blockade. It has already been discussed that there are different dopamine pathways in the brain and that each of those pathways has different roles. Some of those pathways are thought to function normally in schizophrenia (the nigrostriatal and tuberoinfundibular pathways), while others are either overproducing dopamine or not producing enough dopamine. The typical antipsychotics do not affect dopamine receptors in any specified way, so they will attach to D2 receptors in all pathways in the brain and cause a decrease in dopamine overall. So, in the mesolimbic pathway in schizophrenia it is thought to overproduce dopamine, which leads to positive psychotic symptoms. When a typical antipsychotic is used, which blocks dopamine at those D2 receptors, it decreases dopamine in the mesolimbic pathway and leads to a decrease in positive psychotic symptoms, one of the main goals of antipsychotics. However, there are other effects seen based on the antipsychotics' mechanism in the other pathways. The negative symptoms of schizophrenia, characterized by decreased activity, lack of drive, and lack of pleasure, the opposite behaviors that dopamine promotes, are thought to be caused by a baseline lower level of dopamine in the mesocortical dopaminergic pathway. A typical antipsychotic will not be able to avoid targeting the receptors in this pathway, so it will attach to the D2 receptors of the mesocortical pathway leading to an even further decrease in dopamine in that part of the brain, which is thought to lead to the worsening cognitive and negative symptoms often seen with people taking antipsychotics. Neither the nigrostriatal pathway nor the tuberoinfundibular pathway is thought to be altered in schizophrenia or psychotic disorders. So, if a person is suffering from a psychotic disorder, it is thought that while the dopamine is increased in the mesolimbic pathway and decreased in the mesocortical pathway, their dopamine levels in the other two pathways should be the same as a person without a psychotic disorder. But again, the typical antipsychotics are not able to differentiate between D2 receptors, so they attach to receptors in both the nigrostriatal and tuberoinfundibular pathways and lead to a decrease in dopamine in both of those pathways. Recall that the nigrostriatal pathway is largely involved with voluntary movements. So a decrease of dopamine in this pathway can lead to a change in movements, called extrapyramidal movements, which are involuntary and can be distressing. These will be discussed further when discussing side effects of the medications. Similarly, the effect in the tuberoinfundibular pathway can lead to an unwanted side effect. Dopamine acts as an inhibitor to prolactin; so when dopamine is decreased, it can lead to an increase in prolactin which can cause unwanted side effects that will be discussed later. So, overall blockade of D2 receptors in all pathways without ability to specify pathway or receptor type is the way that all typical antipsychotics impact dopamine levels in the brain. As mentioned in an earlier chapter, the main difference in mechanism of action of the typical antipsychotics is how potent they are and how strongly they are attracted to and attached to the dopamine receptors. On the other hand, the atypical antipsychotics have a slightly more complicated role with dopamine and are not such a uniformly understood class of medications.

How Atypical Antipsychotics Affect Dopamine

The atypical antipsychotics are more complicated than the typical antipsychotics, and the complexities of their mechanisms of action are not completely understood. If you take a few steps back and look at their effect on dopamine, it appears similar to the typical antipsychotics. Because, in general, the atypical antipsychotics also block, or antagonize, dopamine receptors, and many of them do it at the D2 receptor primarily. But as you begin to look closer, the many differences can be seen, but it is still not clear exactly how this impacts the disorder or side effects. One of the differences that can be seen is that while the typical antipsychotics are clearly classified by low, mid, and high potency to distinguish the drugs from one another, there is more variation in each individual medication in the atypical category and no specific classification. For the purposes of this book we will cover them in generalities as opposed to giving details about each individual medication. All of the atypical antipsychotics block some dopamine. While the typical antipsychotics all block D2 receptors, some of the atypical antipsychotics block D2 receptors primarily, but others favor various different receptors ranging from D1 to D5. This difference may have some impact on efficacy as well as side effects as the various receptors are located in higher or lower frequency in different parts of the brain and different pathways. The atypical antipsychotics have also been shown to bind more loosely and dissociate more easily than the typical antipsychotics. This is hypothesized to impact the side effect profile of the atypical antipsychotics. It is thought that the movement side effects, caused by a decrease in dopamine in the nigrostriatal pathway from the antipsychotics, are less prominent or prevalent with atypical antipsychotic use and are hypothesized that this may be because of the ability for the atypicals to dissociate more easily from dopamine receptors. Thus far, the differences between the two classes of medications have been somewhat subtle, and the overall message is that antipsychotics block dopamine in the brain and that is how they cause their therapeutic and side effects. However, some of the atypical antipsychotics are also partial dopamine agonists, meaning that they lead to a decrease in dopamine in certain parts of the brain and cause an increase in dopamine in other parts of the brain. It is not clear exactly how this impacts the treatment of psychotic disorders, and the details of its impact on the specific receptors and pathways are beyond the scope of this book, but it is thought that this may lead to a decrease in positive psychotic symptoms, with a decrease in dopamine in the mesolimbic tract and increase in dopamine in the mesocortical tract, leading to a reduction of negative symptoms. The other major way that atypical antipsychotics differ from typical antipsychotics is that all of them also act on serotonin receptors. This shows how the development of medication changes with this evolution of the schizophrenia hypothesis. Serotonin, its role in psychotic disorders, and how it is affected by antipsychotics will be discussed in the following pages.

Serotonin

Serotonin is a neurotransmitter that is actually found primarily in the gut. It is also found in platelets and in the central nervous system. Outside of the central nervous system it plays a role in many important functions, including gut motility, bone metabolism, organ development, and promotion of cardiovascular growth factor. Like many neurotransmitters it serves a variety of purposes for the body in a large range of different sites; however, for the purposes of this book we will focus on its role in the central nervous system.

Serotonin is created from the amino acid L-tryptophan. It requires two biochemical steps to occur with different enzymes, the first being tryptophan hydroxylase and the second is aromatic amino acid decarboxylase. The first enzyme hydroxylates or adds a hydroxyl (OH) to the amino acid, and this step is the rate-limiting step in the production of serotonin. Next it is decarboxylated by the second enzyme, which means that a carboxyl group is removed and carbon dioxide (CO_2) is released. The final product is serotonin, or 5-hydroxytryptamine (5-HT). Serotonin itself cannot reach the brain because it does not cross the blood brain barrier, so taking an oral serotonin supplement would increase the neurotransmitter in the rest of your body but not alter its presence in your brain. The amino acids that it is made from are able to cross the barrier however and reach the brain. Unlike dopamine, serotonin does not have specifically defined pathways in the brain like the four dopaminergic pathways; it simply has groups of different types of receptors located throughout the brain.

Serotonin Pathways and Functions

The principal site of release of serotonin is from the neurons of the raphe nuclei, which are located in the brain stem. The brain stem is at the back of the brain and adjoins the brain to the spinal cord. It houses the cranial nerves that provide the main motor and sensory innervation to the face and neck. It also plays a very important role in the regulation of cardiac and respiratory functioning, maintains consciousness, regulates the sleep cycle, and controls many basic functions like heart rate, breathing, and eating. The main roles of the raphe nuclei are to house and release serotonin to the rest of the brain. From there, the neurotransmitter travels to various receptors located throughout the brain. These receptors throughout the brain bind serotonin and are not only understood to play a large role in mood regulation but also thought to play a role in modulating sleep, appetite, and some cognitive functions, including memory and learning. While the dopamine pathways project mostly from the middle of the brain toward the frontal lobes, the serotonin receptors are located throughout the brain and their projections are much more widespread in the brain. Like dopamine, serotonin has a number of different receptors. The receptors are broken down into categories from 5-HT1 through 5-HT7, and some of those categories have subcategories of 5-HT1a, 5-HT1b, and so on. Each of these receptor categories and subcategories has slightly different roles and different locations of prevalence in the brain or body, but an understanding of all of them is beyond the scope of this book. Understanding serotonin's potential role in psychiatric disorders is the next step in understanding its role in antipsychotics, and the prevalent receptor types will be discussed further there.

How Psychiatric Disorders Affect Serotonin

The role of serotonin in various psychiatric disorders has been suggested for some time, but the specifics about which psychiatric disorders and the details of its role and impact have varied with time. In the 1950s, the chemical structure of serotonin was being studied and was found to be similar to the chemical structure of some hallucinogens like lysergic acid diethylamide (LSD). LSD is structurally similar to serotonin, and the body confuses it for serotonin. It is able to attach to receptors over serotonin as it has a greater attraction to the receptors than serotonin does. Once it attaches it does not transfer any further information via the receptors and therefore creates an environment that has a decrease in serotonin. From this information it was hypothesized that psychotic disorders may also be caused by a deficiency in serotonin. This hypothesis did not become popular until after the development of clozapine, which is used in treatment-resistant schizophrenia. Clozapine works not only by inhibiting dopamine but also by inhibiting certain serotonin pathways. Because of this and because it was such an effective medication, the serotonin hypothesis gained popularity, but as medications were developed and thought to be effective, the hypothesis also changed with time. In the 1950s, it was also suggested that serotonin played a role in just maintaining normal mental processes. This was established by experiments that tampered with regular serotonin levels and led to behavioral and psychiatric changes in humans and lab animals that resembled the process of naturally occurring mental illnesses. It was therefore concluded that serotonin must play a role in maintaining "normal" mental health.

Serotonin and structures similar to it were being studied for a variety of nonpsychiatric illnesses and disorders around this time. While studying structurally similar compounds it was found that when using these structures, they would bind to serotonin sites and not allow serotonin to bind; they were essentially serving as serotonin antagonists, which would lead to a depressive state in human subjects. And thus, the theory that a decrease in serotonin would lead to depression was developed. This may seem a little confusing, as originally, when these theories were being developed, depression and psychosis were thought to be caused by a decrease in serotonin, by similar mechanisms. However, looking forward, the serotonin hypothesis for psychosis became popular after clozapine was noted to be so effective, and clozapine stood out from the typical antipsychotics because it acts as a serotonin antagonist, inhibiting serotonin. But previously, it was thought that psychotic symptoms occurred with LSD because LSD blocked serotonin receptors, inhibiting serotonin, and this does not quite fit together. As has been discussed previously, the evolution and understanding of psychiatric illnesses and treatments have been complicated and not always well understood. While many were suggesting in the 1950s that structures like LSD were acting as serotonin antagonists, there were other studies suggesting that LSD acted in a serotonin-like manner; instead of antagonizing serotonin, it would be acting as a serotonin replacement, an agonist. This leads to two conflicting theories about how serotonin might be involved in psychotic illnesses. At that time there were theories and some evidence pointing in both directions, and the conclusion was simply that serotonin must be involved in some manner, but how it was involved remained to be seen.

As time has gone on, with the development of new medications, in particular clozapine, and further studies, the serotonin hypothesis has developed, and it is now widely thought that an excess of serotonin plays some role in the presentation of psychotic disorders. It is not believed that serotonin is the only neurotransmitter at play. Hypotheses of psychotic disorders still include an alteration in the normal levels of dopamine along with the levels of serotonin. More and more there is research being put into other neurotransmitters and their potential role in psychotic disorders as well. Decades ago there was focus on one main neurotransmitter, dopamine, and as time goes on, there seems to be more and more evidence that other compounds are at play as well, but instead of replacing the dopamine theory, the general trend is to add more complexity to that theory. As more weight has been put into the serotonin theory of schizophrenia, the medications have changed to address this. The following pages will take a look at how the antipsychotics impact serotonin levels and lead to effective or ineffective treatment.

How Antipsychotics Affect Serotonin

Notice that in the previous section when discussing the role of antipsychotics with dopamine it was broken down into two sections to discuss the differences between typical and atypical antipsychotics and their role with dopamine. When discussing serotonin and antipsychotics, there is no need to discuss the different categories of antipsychotics, simply because the typical antipsychotics have no role with serotonin. As mentioned previously, the typical antipsychotics target dopamine for their effectiveness, and most of their side effects come from effects on dopamine, histamine, and acetylcholine, which will be discussed in a later chapter. The atypical antipsychotics, on the other hand, all have some kind of impact on serotonin. This is the main difference between the two classes of medication, which is interesting to look at through a historical and theoretical perspective. As has been mentioned in earlier pages, the theory of psychotic psychiatric illnesses has developed over time. Initially it only pinpointed dopamine as a potential source of imbalance leading to psychotic disorders, and this theory went hand in hand with the development and distribution of the typical antipsychotics. As theories continued to evolve, the medications were effective but not effective enough, and further research was done and the idea that an imbalance of serotonin may also be playing a role in the psychotic disorders became more prevalent. This went hand in hand with the development and production of atypical antipsychotics. Although the main difference between the two classes is their effect on serotonin, they have similarities as well. As mentioned earlier, the atypical antipsychotics all have some effect on dopamine, most blocking dopamine at the D2 receptors with a few also working as partial agonists on dopamine. Generally speaking, all atypical antipsychotics work by binding to and blocking serotonin at some of their receptors.

It is still unclear exactly how, why, or if the atypical antipsychotics are more effective and/or have less side effects than the typical antipsychotics. One of the reasons why it is felt they might be is because while they continue to bind and block dopamine, most of them seem to bind more tightly to (have a greater affinity for) their serotonin receptors than the dopamine receptors, meaning that their main mechanism of action might be on serotonin while still getting some benefit from their action on dopamine. There are many different types of serotonin receptors, but the category that seems to be most involved in antipsychotic properties is the 5-HT2 category, more specifically the 5-HT2a subtype. This category of receptor initially gained interest as a target for treatment when studies were being done with LSD, because this is the receptor type that LSD was binding to. The distribution of the 5-HT2a receptors further supports their potential role in psychotic disorders as they are densely expressed in the area of the brain where the incoming messages from the cortical and subcortical parts of the brain are being sent to be integrated, which is an area that is implicated in psychosis. While nearly all of the atypical antipsychotics bind to these types of receptors and lead to an inhibition of serotonin there, they all bind with different levels of affinity (attraction), which may impact the varied differences in efficacy and side effect profiles seen between agents in the same class. Most of the atypical antipsychotics also have some type of serotonin agonism, increasing serotonin at certain receptors. The receptor most noted to be targeted for agonist properties is the 5-HT1 receptor category, and agonist action here is thought to produce many of the same therapeutic effects that are seen by antagonism at the 5-HT2 category of receptors.

Like the typical and atypical antipsychotics' interactions with dopamine, the atypical interactions with serotonin are complicated. Their mechanisms of action are partially understood, and the reason that they have therapeutic efficacy becomes more difficult to understand as you look at the specifics of the mechanism and the potential cause of the disorders. Overall, what is generally understood is that atypical antipsychotics all have an inhibiting effect on serotonin at certain receptors, and most have a partial agonist effect at some receptors, meaning that atypical antipsychotics decrease serotonin in some areas and increase serotonin in other areas. It is thought that this activity leads to a reduction in psychotic symptoms which is why the atypical antipsychotics have been effective in treating psychotic disorders as well as bipolar disorder.

Both typical and atypical antipsychotics have some effect in reducing positive psychotic symptoms and maybe some negative psychotic symptoms through their actions on dopamine and serotonin; however, there is still room for improvement. By looking at history one can imagine where things will be headed in the future. In the past there were theories, and medications developed out of these theories. As it was noticed that the theories were not capturing the whole disease, they developed and changed, adding more neurotransmitters to the theory of the disease. This trend seems to be continuing with more compounds being studied and suggested as contributors to the pathophysiology of psychotic disorders.

OTHER POTENTIAL TARGETS

This will be discussed briefly here and in more detail in a later chapter about the future of antipsychotics. Thus far, most of the Food and Drug Administration (FDA)-approved medications target only the two previously mentioned neurotransmitters, dopamine and serotonin. But still psychotic disorders are not treated completely, and all symptoms are not resolved. And so, the hypothesis for the cause of the disorder evolves as well as the potential targets for medications. Perhaps the cause, and thus the treatment, needs to be broader than simply dopamine and serotonin. Acetylcholine, glutamate, and gamma-aminobutyric acid (GABA) are all neurotransmitters that are currently being studied as potential targets. Most of them have been considered potential targets for many years, but in the past decade or so there seems to be more of a push to develop medications that treat psychosis as a whole. And so the possibility that some of these may be developed into medications used to treat psychosis seems to be becoming more of a reality. More recently there have even been theories about compounds that are not neurotransmitters, like oxytocin and histamine, and their potential role in psychosis and their potential as targets for treatment are being studied. As the hypothesis of psychosis is further expanded and more medications are studied, it is unclear what medications will actually be called antipsychotics, how they will be classified, and what other medications might be developed to target some of the other symptoms of psychotic disorders. Likely the understanding of the illnesses and their potential targets for treatment will get more complicated before they become simplified; still it is encouraging that there are many avenues for further development at this time. Even the information we have thus far can be somewhat complicated, so the next few pages will recap what has been covered in this chapter thus far—how the antipsychotics work in the body and impact neurotransmitters and how that may cause a therapeutic effect in psychotic disorders.

Psychiatric illnesses are not completely understood, which makes it difficult to completely understand the mechanism of action and therapeutic efficacy of the medications used to treat them. Antipsychotics thus far target neurotransmitters, specifically dopamine and serotonin, in order to cause a decrease in psychotic symptoms. But neurotransmitters are complicated and categorized and have a variety of pathways that cannot always be specified by medications, and, therefore, many side effects and unwanted effects ensue. Typical antipsychotics work by decreasing dopamine. Atypical antipsychotics work by both decreasing and increasing dopamine as well as decreasing and increasing serotonin. And still these medications do not usually lead to a complete resolution of symptoms, at least in the person with a chronic psychotic disorder. These statements are simple, but the application of the medications is complex. In the following chapters, we will explore what effects the medications actually have and how they are applied, which leads to an exploration of the nontherapeutic effects or side effects and risk of misuse of the medications. This further exploration of how the medications work and how they are applied in clinical settings sheds more light and understanding on the complexities of the diseases they are meant to treat and mechanisms of action targeted to treat them.

Chapter 5

Effects and Applications

At this point you have a general understanding of what antipsychotics are, how they were developed, and how they actually work at a chemical level, with an idea of some of the effects they may cause. But in order to really understand how they can have an impact, you must understand the specifics of both the therapeutic effects and adverse effects that they can cause. Thus far, in the book, the focus has been on schizophrenia, as it is a classic example of a psychotic disorder that would require antipsychotics for treatment. However, there are many different psychiatric and medical illnesses that have a psychotic component leading to antipsychotics as the choice of treatment. This chapter will explore the different effects that can be seen when using antipsychotics, with a focus on the therapeutic effects, as the adverse effects will be covered in detail later on. It will also discuss not only what effects the medications have but also how well they actually work and for what kind of illnesses they are indicated for.

THERAPEUTIC EFFECTS OF ANTIPSYCHOTICS

As one might assume simply after considering the name of this category of medications that they in fact work against psychosis, which is exactly correct. That is somewhat of an oversimplification, however, and the medications and their effects are much more complex than that. In order to understand what their therapeutic effects would be, you must first have an understanding of what some of the unwanted symptoms are. As psychotic symptoms are the clear target of these medications, it makes sense to start with them. To review some of the psychotic symptoms already mentioned in this book, they can broadly be divided into positive and negative symptoms. The positive symptoms are the symptoms that can be most easily identified by outside observers and are often considered most distressing by external sources. The negative symptoms can often be easily overlooked by outside observers. They involve a change in a person's ability to think clearly, to plan and execute tasks, and to be motivated. They also impact a person's ability to express emotion. These symptoms, while easily overlooked by the outsider, often have a much greater impact on an individual's overall functioning. Both aspects of psychosis can be distressing in different ways, and different types are seen in different psychotic diseases, which will be discussed later on. But first, what kind of changes can be seen in a person who suffers from some positive symptoms of psychosis when they begin taking an antipsychotic?

Positive Symptoms

The three broad categories of positive symptoms are delusions, perceptual disturbances, and thought disorders. Antipsychotics have some type of effect on all of these; however, their effectiveness varies between categories of positive symptoms. As this book has explored various aspects of antipsychotics, it has become clear that antipsychotics and the illnesses they treat are complex, and there is still much more to be learned about the diseases and the medications. There is still a lot that is not known about what causes psychosis, although we have already covered some long-standing and some newer hypotheses that give an understanding of how some of the symptoms may be caused. Similarly, there are aspects of antipsychotics and their mechanism of action that are understood and that fit into the hypotheses of psychosis, but there are aspects of both the medications and the diseases that are not clearly understood. If it were as simple as psychosis being caused by too much dopamine and antipsychotics working as dopamine blockers, then it could be hypothesized that if you gave someone with symptoms of psychosis an antipsychotic, all of their psychotic symptoms would remit and they would return to what their baseline was. However, as one might guess, it is more complicated than that, and as was covered in the previous chapter, there are multiple different neurotransmitters that are thought to be involved and multiple different pathways for the neurotransmitters that complicate both the disease process and the therapeutic process. In order to try to make this material more digestible, the following paragraphs will explore positive psychotic symptoms, how they are thought to be produced, and what kind of effects antipsychotics are thought to have upon them.

The positive symptoms of psychosis are generally thought to be produced by an excess of dopamine in the brain. All antipsychotics act to block some amount of dopamine in the brain and therefore produce a decrease in some of the positive symptoms of psychosis. Antipsychotics seem to work better on some positive symptoms than others, but the overall effect is to cause a reduction in positive psychotic symptoms. But as mentioned earlier, they do not work perfectly; they have different results for different individuals and for different types of positive symptoms. What could one expect to see when a person suffering from positive symptoms of psychosis is started on an antipsychotic? Typically you can expect a reduction in the positive symptoms within the first week of starting the medication, but it may take several weeks to reach their full effect. It is also not typical that positive psychotic symptoms will be completely eliminated. It is more likely that the symptoms will become less frequent, less intense, and/or less distressing to the individual; however, it is likely that some of the positive symptoms will continue. To get a better idea of how this might look in the real world, the next few paragraphs will look at some clinical scenarios of how symptoms might be changed after starting an antipsychotic.

As an example, Charles is a 28-year-old male who comes to the psychiatrist's office for an initial appointment. During the first appointment, he tells the doctor that he graduated from law school three years ago, and about one year prior he got a job working at a reputable law firm that he hopes to make partner at one day. Things have been going alright there, but he is under a lot of stress and pressure and has been working very long hours. He says that the first six months there went really well but then things started to catch up to him a little bit, and he has been struggling to stay ahead and get his work done lately. He says for the past three to four weeks he has not been feeling like himself and has been struggling to motivate himself to do things. He is starting to feel like he is just a failure and will always be a failure. For the past three weeks, he has missed some work and is not hanging out with his friends or coworkers anymore. He also states that he has been having a very difficult time sleeping and has been so upset about work that he just does not feel like eating much anymore. Lastly, he states that for the past two weeks he has started to hear a voice, sometimes two. He says they come at random times throughout the day, and he does not seem to be able to control when they come or when they stop. When asked what they usually say, he is hesitant to reply at first and then states that they do not say very nice things. He says that sometimes they just tell him what a failure he is and how he will never become anything, and other times it is worse. He did not think he really needed to see anyone about them as he thought they would go away on their own when his stress would decrease, but when they started telling him he should just give up and jump off a roof he became concerned and decided to try to get some help. The psychiatrist talks to him about a group of medications called antipsychotics that he thinks could help with the auditory hallucinations that he is having. He also feels that he should start an antidepressant to help improve his mood and return in a week to see how the medications are working.

Charles agrees with the plan. He begins taking the antipsychotic and the antidepressant and returns in a week. When he comes back, he reports that he has been taking his medication every day, and while he is still occasionally hearing the voices, they are coming much less frequently, and he states that they are easier to ignore than they used to be. Over the past few days he has heard them only every other day and for just a few minutes when they come, as opposed to before when he was hearing them multiple times a day for up to a half an hour at a time. He discusses this with the psychiatrist and is happy to learn that he is showing a good response to the medication and that with time the hallucinations will likely become less frequent. He also states that in his case if he continues to take the antidepressant and has improvement in his mood, it is possible that all of his symptoms will go into remission.

In the scenario above, the patient is showing symptoms of a depressed mood with psychotic symptoms. He is experiencing auditory hallucinations with his symptoms of depression. The psychiatrist recognizes that, so offers a medication to treat his mood, the antidepressant, and a medication to treat his positive psychotic symptoms, an antipsychotic. The patient begins taking it and has a decrease in the frequency of his auditory hallucinations. As mentioned above, it is expected if the patient is responding to the antipsychotic, then there will be a reduction in symptoms in the first week, but it may take several weeks to show full effect. In some diseases it is unlikely that the symptoms will be eliminated entirely, but in others it is expected. In a disease like the one in the previous case, major depression with psychotic features, it is expected that if both the depressive symptoms and psychotic symptoms are effectively addressed, the individual can have complete remission of all symptoms. This however varies from disease to disease and will be addressed throughout the following pages and chapters as different diseases come up.

Auditory hallucinations are one of three different types of positive psychotic symptoms. Delusions can be present in different disease processes and are another positive symptom. Take for example, Mary, a 32-year-old female who was admitted to a psychiatric hospital after she came to the emergency department with her husband, Ray, who said that she had not been sleeping lately, had not been acting like herself, and was saying all sorts of strange things. When the psychiatrist meets her for the first time, she is wearing a neon green sweatshirt with jeans and a polka dot skirt over them. She has multiple necklaces on and has her hair pulled back in three different braids. She begins speaking rapidly, switching from topic to topic. She talks about how she has never felt this good before and has been able to get so much done since she has been in the hospital. She is happy to remark how she is amazed that she is feeling so good and does not even need to sleep anymore! The psychiatrist is hardly even able to get a word in as she tells him about all of the different things she has been doing and plans to do. She begins telling him about how before she came in she was working on some music that she had started writing. She continues on to tell him that she is a famous songwriter as well as a lawyer and actress. When the doctor tries to ask her a few questions about what she has been doing at home, she continues on to talk about how she has met and is friends with the president of the United States and the Queen of England. She states that the president is often asking for her advice about diplomatic dilemmas. After a lengthy conversation with the psychiatrist and Ray, she agrees to take a medication, an antipsychotic, that may make her feel more like her normal self. The medication is started and since she is hospitalized and can be monitored regularly, it can be increased more rapidly than as an outpatient. After about two to three days of taking the antipsychotic, she begins to get a little more sleep at night and is speaking more slowly. At this time if you ask her directly if she knows the president or the Queen of England, she states that she does. But she no longer brings it up herself, and she does not go on to elaborate about their relationship. She continues to write her song lyrics but does not discuss them unless asked. Mary continues to take the antipsychotic, and after about nine days she is feeling much more like herself. She no longer believes that she has a relationship with the president of the United States or the Queen of England. And while she enjoys listening to music and is thinking about taking some guitar lessons, she no longer thinks she is a songwriter or actress and feels that she is almost ready to go back to her work as a journalist.

In the above vignette, Mary presents to the emergency department with symptoms of acute mania with psychosis. It is common for individuals in acute mania to have positive symptoms of psychosis, and acute mania responds well to antipsychotic treatment. Mary came in with grandiose delusions of having multiple professions (songwriter, lawyer, actress) and having close relationships with world leaders. After starting her antipsychotic, she quickly, but gradually, showed an improvement in her grandiose delusions. First they become less externally apparent. She still believes these delusions, but they are less powerful and overbearing to her, so she does not readily discuss them. She also may know at that point that some people may find what she is saying a bit odd. This change can occur within the first few days and should be seen within the first week. Beyond that the antipsychotics continue to work and will show a fuller effect over the next few weeks. Mary, by the time of discharge from the hospital, no longer has her grandiose ideas about her relationships and career. The psychotic symptoms that occur with acute mania can be treated by antipsychotics and achieve full remission. Antipsychotics are often used during the acute phase of mania when positive psychotic symptoms are most noticeable, and as improvements are made, the antipsychotic is some-times continued with a mood stabilizer and other times is replaced by a mood stabilizer. Again, while some psychotic symptoms are difficult to completely eliminate, it is often the case that when psychotic symptoms are part of the manic phase of bipolar disorder, they can be completely remitted by antipsy-chotics and stabilization of mood.

The other aspect of positive psychotic symptoms is the thought process and the disorganization that can come with psychosis. For example, James is a 43-year-old man with a history of mental illness. In the past he has been on an antipsychotic, but he stopped taking it a few years back and had been doing pretty well for some time. In the past month his family has noticed that some-times he is not making much sense when he talks, and at their urging he agreed to come to the psychiatrist's office. When he meets the psychiatrist, he tells him that he feels okay but that he does not feel quite like himself. He says that he feels like his thoughts have been difficult to get out, and sometimes his mind feels clouded or jumbled. The psychiatrist notices that when he speaks his rate and rhythm are normal, but he is using words that do not make sense. He answers questions inappropriately and at times stops in the middle of a sen-tence as if he forgot he was in the middle of a conversation. For instance, when asking him about his past psychiatric treatment, James begins by stating that he used to get care at the building with the windows that was near his old work and then continues on to talk about his past job and education, but he never answers the question and he makes illogical statements when talking. In the middle of talking about his past work, he pauses for about 35 seconds and does not continue with the conversation until the psychiatrist reminds him of the question. At the end of the session the psychiatrist talks with James about his current difficulty with his thoughts and integrating them into his speech. He suggests that he start back on an antipsychotic as this could be a symptom of his mental illness that would respond well to antipsychotics. James agrees with this treatment and begins taking an antipsychotic. He returns to the clinic in one week and reports that he is feeling a little clearer, but family members state that at times he still does not make sense. It seems he is having a small response to the medication, so the dose is increased and he returns home. At his follow-up appointment two weeks later he is pleased to report that his mind is feeling much less cloudy, and he thinks his speech is making more sense. His family members agree that he has much improved since starting the medication, and while he is close to his baseline, he is still not quite all the way back to normal.

In the clinical scenario above, James presents to an outpatient psychiatrist after stopping his antipsychotic medication years earlier. He is having symptoms of the third type of positive psychotic symptoms, thought disorders. And as is often the case with the positive psychotic symptoms, it was noticed by his family members. He is presenting with disorganized thoughts and some thought blocking. James cannot identify exactly what is wrong, but he can tell that he is not thinking as clearly as he normally does. Thought disorders are quite varied in their presentation. His presentation is likely most consistent with schizophrenia. In the case of schizophrenia and thought disorders, as opposed to the two previous examples, it is likely that there will be an improvement with the organization of the thoughts when taking antipsychotics, but often there is not a complete remission of symptoms. Antipsychotics will help diminish the severity of the thought disorder, and other modalities of treatment can be utilized to help with more complete remission of symptoms.

The three scenarios above provide a general understanding of how antipsychotics can lead to improvement in positive psychotic symptoms. If an individual shows response to a particular antipsychotic, he or she will show a reduction in psychotic symptoms; however, the extent of remission of positive psychotic symptoms often depends on what disorder is causing them. Antipsychotics' role with positive psychotic symptoms is quite clear and has been demonstrated in many studies; on the other hand, their effect on the negative symptoms of psychosis is not as obvious and is considered more complicated as discussed next.

Negative Symptoms

As was discussed earlier in the book, while it is thought that the positive symptoms are caused by an increase in dopamine, specifically in the mesolimbic tract, it is thought that negative symptoms are often caused by a decrease in dopamine in the mesocortical tract. Some of the older research that supports this theory is based on studies of patients with schizophrenia who were already being treated with a phenothiazine. Recall that phenothiazines are the base chemical structure for some of the earliest typical antipsychotics. These patients were given L-dopa and were found to have statistically significant improvements in symptoms. Initially that sounds like it may work against the working hypotheses on excess dopamine causing positive psychotic symptoms and depletion of dopamine causing negative psychotic symptoms. However, the improvements that were seen were not in positive psychotic symptoms; they saw an improvement in patients who had lost spontaneity and had lack of initiative and apathy. They found an improvement in negative symptoms with administration of L-dopa. It is fitting with the hypothesis that the positive psychotic symptoms are secondary to an increase in dopamine, and the negative psychotic symptoms are secondary to a decrease in dopamine. In those patients that had positive psychotic symptoms, they were being treated with an antipsychotic, decreasing dopamine in certain parts of the brain. By supplementing with L-dopa, one is causing an increase in dopamine, at least in a certain part of the brain, that provides relief and improvement in some of the negative symptoms.

All antipsychotics block dopamine, which serves to help decrease the positive symptoms but can worsen negative symptoms. As has been discussed, while the positive symptoms are distressing and easily noticed by external observers, it is often the negative symptoms that cause a major impact on long-term functioning. For that reason, a focus of antipsychotic research has been on developing antipsychotics that can be more specific and target other receptors in order to lead to an improvement in negative symptoms. Unfortunately, currently there are not many antipsychotics that cause a large reduction in negative symptoms, and some cause them to worsen.

The typical antipsychotics are all strong dopamine antagonists, and this serves as their main neurotransmitter interaction. For that reason, most of the typical antipsychotics either do not influence or end up worsening negative symptoms. The atypical antipsychotics still not only block dopamine, but they also work on other transmitters, namely serotonin, and do not have high affinity toward dopamine receptors. This might lead to their increased ability to reduce negative symptoms; at least that was part of the hope in their development. The hope in developing the atypical antipsychotics is multifold. When developing new medications, it is always the goal to make them more specific, making them more effective with fewer side effects. For antipsychotics, the goal is to develop newer drugs that target both positive and negative psychotic symptoms with fewer side effects, especially motor side effects. Whether or not they were effective as better drugs was debated and continues to be debated; however, they are still used much more frequently over typical antipsychotics, with the belief that they have greater benefits with lower risks. There was a well-known National Institute of Mental Health (NIMH)-funded clinical study that aimed to compare the effectiveness of the typical antipsychotics with the atypical antipsychotics. The trial is called the Clinical Antipsychotic Trials of Intervention Effectiveness (CATIE) study and is the largest, longest, and most comprehensive independent trial studying therapies for schizophrenia. The goal of this trial was to compare the two classes and help to guide daily clinical treatment decisions. The study looked at three atypical antipsychotics (olanzapine, risperidone, and quetiapine) and one typical antipsychotic (perphenazine) and lasted 18 months. Ziprasidone, another atypical antipsychotic, was added later on in the study after it was approved by the Food and Drug Administration (FDA). The primary measure of treatment success in the study was how long a patient stayed on a medication with the idea that the medication is critical to controlling symptoms and preventing relapse. The study found that overall the medications were comparably effective but that all of them were associated with high rates of discontinuation. Overall, 74% of patients discontinued the medications before the 18 months were complete. Olanzapine, one of the atypical antipsychotics, was slightly better as far as percentage of patients who dropped out of the study, but it was associated with significant weight gain as a side effect. The older, typical antipsychotic, perphenazine, generally performed as well as the atypical antipsychotics. The study showed that movement side effects were not more common in the typical compared to the atypical antipsychotics as was expected. While it remains unclear how these results should impact clinical decision making, it has made it clear that there is much more progress to be made with antipsychotics or perhaps a different class of medication, particularly to attempt to address side effects and the negative symptoms of psychosis.

The prior few pages discussed how antipsychotics may have an effect upon both positive and negative psychotic symptoms, and the focus thus far in the book has been on antipsychotics' impact on psychotic symptoms. However, they have been shown to be effective in managing other symptoms as well. One of the better studied behavioral symptoms that antipsychotics have been shown to impact is impulsive aggression.

Impulsive Aggression

Impulsive aggression is characterized by inability to regulate affect and aggressive impulses. As one could imagine, this can become quite dangerous for the individual who is unable to regulate these impulses as well as others around that individual. An inability to regulate one's affect also gives an internal feeling of being out of control, which can be very distressing to a person. Impulsive aggression is highly comorbid with other psychiatric illnesses. Biochemical, brain imaging, and genetic studies have suggested that dysfunctional interactions between serotonin and dopamine, specifically in the prefrontal cortex, are an important mechanism underlying this link between the aggression and comorbid disorders. It is thought that a decrease in serotonin, or its functioning, and an increase in dopamine are two of the major components predisposing individuals to impulsive aggression. As we know, typical antipsychotics work to block dopamine in various areas of the brain, including the prefrontal cortex, which would lead one to believe they may be beneficial in managing impulsive aggression. Similarly, some of the atypical antipsychotics, in particular the newer atypicals, work in multiple ways. Some of the newer ones block dopamine and work as both serotonin agonists and antagonists, meaning that they block serotonin at certain subtypes of serotonin receptors and they increase serotonin at other subtypes of serotonin receptors. One could imagine how this would be useful in working toward managing an individual's impulsive aggression.

To get a clearer picture of what this might look like clinically, take for example George, who is a 10-year-old boy with autism spectrum disorder. His parents have been working with multiple different specialties throughout his life to help him function outside of the home and remain safe. They have been working with speech and language specialists, behavioral specialists, and a psychiatrist. They come to visit the psychiatrist for a monthly visit and state that over the past two to three months his aggression and irritability have gotten worse. They are beginning to get more concerned about him as he gets older and bigger because they are worried that he can cause more damage and may cause more harm to himself. Usually when something does not go his way or when there is a change in his very strict and regimented routine, he gets very upset. He used to just cry out and rock back and forth, but now he is starting to hit himself in the head or sometimes bang his head against the wall, and his parents are unable to stop this behavior. Together with the psychiatrist they decide to try aripiprazole, one of the atypical antipsychotics, as it has been shown to be effective in reducing this type of aggressive and irritable behavior. They return to the clinic three weeks later stating that things have been improving at home. Of course George still gets upset when his routine is altered, but the parents have found that he is hitting himself much less frequently, and they are able to provide him comfort more easily when he seems to be in distress.

The clinical scenario above demonstrates how an atypical antipsychotic may produce therapeutic effects when targeting behavioral disturbances of impulsive aggression and irritability. This behavior is common in autism spectrum disorder and can be quite concerning, dangerous, and often difficult to treat. Aripiprazole is one of the antipsychotics that is FDA-approved to be used in this patient population for behavioral disturbances. However, there are behavioral disturbances of aggression and irritability that are comorbid with many of the other psychiatric illnesses and often in special patient populations. Recall from the second chapter that antipsychotics have FDA-approved uses but that many are used "off-label" for other uses too. This means that the medication has not been officially approved for use of that disorder but that the doctor feels it would be medically beneficial and appropriate. Impulsive aggression and irritability are target symptoms that many antipsychotics are used off-label for. This will be discussed in greater detail later in the chapter when discussing indications for antipsychotics in medical use.

The previous pages cover some of the therapeutic effects that may be seen with antipsychotic use. As has been discussed thus far, the mechanism of action of antipsychotics is complex and still not completely understood, making their therapeutic and adverse effects also complex and still not completely understood. The above gives a general overview of the effects that could be expected to be seen but by no means covers all of the effects that may be possible. In earlier chapters, some of the potential side effects have been mentioned but not discussed in detail. As one could imagine since these medications have multiple modes of action and impact various different systems, they have somewhat complex and extensive potential side effect profiles. These risks and adverse effects will be discussed in greater detail in the following chapter. Now that we have covered how the antipsychotics work and what therapeutic effects could be expected, the remainder of the chapter will focus on how effective they are when they are indicated for use and how to use them in special patient populations.

HOW WELL DO ANTIPSYCHOTICS WORK?

Generally in medicine when trying to determine if a medication is efficacious or not, it is helpful to look for objective measures of improvement. For example, if someone has pneumonia and is treated with an antibiotic, in order to determine if the medication is efficacious you initially monitor their temperature (looking for fever) and get a chest x-ray. During treatment you continue to monitor for a decrease in temperature and eventually follow up with a repeat chest x-ray. The chest x-ray and temperature are objective measures to determine that the medication is working and the pneumonia is going away. Similarly, when someone has elevated blood pressure, it is treated with an antihypertensive. After giving the medication, the patient's blood pressure serves as the objective measure to determine how well the antihypertensive is working. This is slightly more complicated with antipsychotics as they are generally trying to achieve a decrease in psychotic symptoms; however, as has been noted already, they are also used for a variety of other functions. Even if just looking at a decrease in psychotic symptoms, this is somewhat of a subjective determination. For that reason there have been scales created to determine the change in psychotic symptoms and therefore the effectiveness of the antipsychotics.

One of the most well-studied and widely used scales of measuring psychotic symptoms is the Positive and Negative Syndrome Scale (PANSS), which was developed out of the need for a well-operationalized method of assessing these symptoms and syndromes. It has been shown to be both a valid and reliable scale and has been used to assess the efficacy of antipsychotic treatment in both research trials as well as clinical practices. It is, as the name describes, a 30-item scale that rates various aspects of a patient's both positive and negative symptoms. If being used in clinical practice, it can be administered at various points throughout treatment with antipsychotics to determine how much improvement a patient is experiencing in different aspects of their symptomatology.

Studies of antipsychotics and their effectiveness have shown that all of the available antipsychotics are clearly more effective than placebo in treating schizophrenia. There is a lack of specific studies on typical antipsychotics examining the effectiveness of them in the many other psychiatric illnesses that they are approved for treating such as schizophreniform, bipolar, or schizoaffective disorders. The atypical antipsychotics have all been studied and shown to be effective for schizophrenia and bipolar disorder. It is important to understand that they are more effective than placebo, so it could be assumed that they are helpful to patients who are suffering from psychotic symptoms. That leads to the question—how effective are they? How much do they help?

It is difficult to answer that question in general because they have different rates of efficacy depending on the individual and the disease that they are being used to treat. It also depends on how you measure efficacy. As mentioned previously, some use rating scales to determine improvement. In clinical practice people often use patient report, and in trials they often determine efficacy by patient discontinuation rate. Studies involving hospitalized patients have shown at least moderate improvement in symptoms in at least 75% of patients. However, most patients never achieve complete remission, making it more difficult to return to the community and function at an independent level. But again, it depends on the disease process that is being treated. For example, antipsychotics in combination with mood stabilizers have been shown to be very effective, particularly in the acutely manic phase of bipolar disorder. While more studies need to be done and probably more effective objective measurements created to determine efficacy of various antipsychotics in different illnesses, there are data that help to predict the percentage of receptors that need to be altered in order for the medication to be efficacious. For an antipsychotic to be effective, it generally requires antagonism of 60–80% of D2 receptors. It has been determined that at lower levels of dopamine antagonism there are no active antipsychotic properties and at levels higher than that more extensive side effects are produced without any extra benefit. This is not to say that for everyone once 60–80% of D2 receptors are antagonized, there will be improvement in symptoms, as some people do not respond to the medications, and others will have some improvement but will continue with symptoms. If an individual is going to respond to the medication, he or she will generally show some improvement in the first few weeks. The majority of improvement is seen within the first six weeks. For most people this is a gradual improvement in symptoms, and while the majority will be seen in the first six weeks, slowly throughout the next few months there could be a continued reduction in symptoms.

This leads to a discussion of the final way that people measure efficacy, by patient discontinuation of medication. It seems that antipsychotics are at least somewhat beneficial in the majority of patients, greater than 75%. For some psychotic diseases the duration of treatment may not be that long; however, for the majority of psychotic illnesses, treatment is recommended for months, to years, to lifelong. Therefore, it would be important for efficacy to have medications that are tolerable for long periods of time. As mentioned previously, in the CATIE trial that primarily looked at discontinuation as an outcome measure, 74% of patients stopped the medication prior to completion of the trial, 18 months. This shows that even if the antipsychotics are effective in reducing symptoms, there is something about them that is not tolerable and therefore causes them to be ineffective in long-term treatment. Researchers and clinicians have understood for some time that the goal should be to develop antipsychotics that are both more effective in reducing symptoms and more tolerable. That has been the goal with the ongoing production and development of atypical antipsychotics. It is questionable, however, how successful that has been. There is one atypical antipsychotic, clozapine, that has been shown to be more efficacious than other typical and atypical antipsychotics; however, it has a dangerous side effect profile.

Clozapine

Clozapine was the first atypical antipsychotic developed and has a more unique profile than any of the other antipsychotics. It has also been shown to be more effective than other antipsychotics in resistant schizophrenia. Clozapine has more D1 than D2 effects than other antipsychotics. Because of this it has more effect on cortical and limbic dopaminergic systems and less on the basal ganglia (motor control), which might be why it is more effective in treating symptoms and has less propensity to cause the movement side effects that are seen with the other antipsychotics. It also has greater serotonergic, histaminic, and alpha adrenergic blocking activity than other antipsychotics. It is unclear if that aspect of its profile has more to do with its effectiveness or its side effect profile, which is also slightly different than the other antipsychotics or a combination of both. There is suggestion that if any of the antipsychotics may assist with improving negative symptoms, it is clozapine. While other antipsychotics require between 60% and 80% of D2 receptors to be antagonized in order to show antipsychotic properties, clozapine shows antipsychotic properties and improvement in symptoms at less than 60% of binding. The difference in effectiveness is not a small one. One of the pivotal trials showing clozapine's greater efficacy found significant improvement in 30% of patients treated with clozapine as compared to improvement in only 5% of patients being treated with chlorpromazine, the first typical antipsychotic. These studies are showing clozapine's effectiveness in the treatment of resistant schizophrenia. There is not good data confirming its efficacy in bipolar or schizoaffective disorders; however, there is some evidence suggesting that it has advantages in both. One of the other interesting aspects of clozapine's effectiveness is that is has been shown to reduce suicidality, meaning suicide attempts and suicidal thinking, in patients with schizophrenia. It has actually been FDA-approved for use to reduce the risk of suicidal behavior in patients with schizophrenia or schizoaffective disorder. All of this information makes it seem like clozapine would be the clear first choice for treating psychosis. However, it is also the most regulated antipsychotic because of its side effect profile.

Clozapine has been in use in Europe for more than 30 years and was withdrawn from general use after deaths from agranulocytosis were reported in the mid-1970s. Agranulocytosis refers to an acute condition involving an extreme decrease in white blood cell count. A very low white blood cell count puts an individual at great risk for infection and eventual death. For this reason, clozapine is heavily regulated in the United States, and that regulation will be discussed in further detail in a later chapter. The rate of agranulocytosis is estimated to be approximately 1% in the United States. The risk of agranulocytosis decreases greatly as the treatment continues, with the period of highest risk considered to be between weeks 4 and 18. Because of this potentially fatal side effect, clozapine is not considered a first-line treatment for psychosis but would cause one to wonder why more medications with similar mechanisms are not developed. Some of the more recent atypical antipsychotics, like olanzapine, have attempted to utilize the basic chemical structure of clozapine and to create comparable mechanisms of action. Unfortunately, none of the newer atypical antipsychotics have been shown to have a similar efficacy to clozapine thus far, and this continues to be an area in need of further research and development.

The previous pages have provided an overview of what kind of effects these medications may cause and how much they may help. Throughout the chapters thus far there has been reference to the different psychiatric disorders that may benefit from antipsychotic treatment, but the next few pages will examine this further, detailing what the medical indications are for antipsychotic treatment.

INDICATIONS FOR MEDICAL USE

In general the indications for antipsychotic use can be broken down into two broad categories: psychotic disorders and psychotic symptoms in other disorders. The psychotic disorders are considered primary psychiatric illnesses, whereas the psychotic symptoms in other disorders could be secondary to medical complications, substances or other psychiatric disorders that are not primarily psychotic in nature.

Psychotic Disorders

Throughout the chapters thus far we have focused on psychotic disorders in general or schizophrenia but have not touched on the specific psychotic disorders where antipsychotics are indicated. Antipsychotics are indicated in most psychotic disorders, as would be expected, but understanding those diseases and how antipsychotics could be useful is important.

Schizophrenia

Schizophrenia is a chronic psychotic disorder characterized by a constellation of both positive and negative psychotic symptoms. The disease can be diagnosed if there are a certain number of both positive and negative symptoms present for at least six months along with significant social or occupational functional impairment. The disease prevalence is about 1%, meaning that it affects approximately 1% of people over their lifetime. People generally begin to start showing symptoms in their 20s or 30s and rarely before 15 or after 55. This is one of the psychiatric illnesses that has been shown to have strong genetic links.

Antipsychotics are the mainstay treatment for schizophrenia. There are other types of therapies that can go along with antipsychotics to target some of the symptoms that impair functioning like cognitive and behavioral therapy, but as far as medications are concerned antipsychotics are the key. It is commonly understood and believed that a person showing psychotic symptoms that meets criteria for the diagnosis of schizophrenia should be started on an antipsychotic. However, this psychiatric illness is somewhat unique in the fact that the illness is thought to have a prodromal phase. This is a period of time that can last months to years before the overt psychotic symptoms are seen. During this period, a person would show a decline in overall functioning, particularly in the social area. They may become more withdrawn and isolated. Some have vague mood symptoms that occur during this time such as anxiety or depression, and they may display some bizarre behaviors or thinking. At this time their symptoms are considered subthreshold, meaning they do not meet criteria for a diagnosis but they are beginning to resemble the schizophrenia picture. In the past one to two decades, this prodromal phase has become an area of great interest in the field of psychiatry, particularly because of possible treatments. It is widely accepted that the duration of untreated psychosis in a person with a first psychotic episode has an impact on the course and prognosis of the person's schizophrenia. The shorter the duration of untreated psychosis, the better the outcome in the short and long term. The focus in the past few decades has been not only on treating once the psychotic episode and the diagnosis of schizophrenia have been established, but the question of prevention has arisen as well. Currently there is no consensus on exactly when to treat people who are considered to be in the prodromal phase or even what to treat them with. Both antipsychotics and antidepressants have been studied, but at this point the results are not clear enough to make a recommendation, as there has been some conflicting research. However, antipsychotics have shown some prospects in the treatment of the prodromal phase of schizophrenia, and it will be interesting to see how the research in this field develops. So currently it is clearly indicated that antipsychotics should be the first-line treatment for schizophrenia, and it remains unclear if they are useful in the prodromal phase of schizophrenia.

Schizoaffective Disorder

Schizoaffective disorder is classified as a psychotic disorder; however, it has a major mood component as well. There are two components to making a diagnosis of schizoaffective disorder. One must have a period of illness that meets criteria for a major mood disorder, either a depressive episode or a manic episode. During that time period, the person must also have at least two psychotic symptoms, including delusions, hallucinations, disorganized speech, grossly disorganized behavior, or negative symptoms. Separate from that period of illness the person must have two weeks of either delusions or hallucinations without mood symptoms (either depression or mania). To simplify, a person must have a period with mood symptoms (either depression or mania) and psychotic symptoms as well as a period of psychotic symptoms without any pathologic mood symptoms. Onset of the disorder is usually in young adulthood, and exact prevalence is not known at this time. It is estimated to be under 1% and likely somewhere between 0.5% and 0.8%. While schizophrenia generally has quite an impact on a person's functioning, the course of schizoaffective disorder can be quite variable. Some do very well with treatment, and others suffer a more chronically debilitating course. Many with the disorder suffer comorbid disorders, specifically anxiety disorders and substance use disorders. Antipsychotics are a necessary part of the treatment of schizoaffective disorder; however, they are not the only medication necessary for treatment. Someone diagnosed with schizoaffective disorder should be started on an antipsychotic and either a mood stabilizer or antidepressant, depending on what type of mood component the person suffers from. In this disorder, the antipsychotic will then target the psychotic symptoms, and the mood stabilizer or antidepressant will target the mood symptoms.

Delusional Disorder

Delusional disorder is somewhat unique when compared to many of the other psychotic disorders or nonpsychotic disorders with psychotic features. It is classified by the presence of one or more delusions for one month or longer. Interestingly, one cannot have other prominent psychotic symptoms. One of the aspects that distinguishes delusional disorder from most other psychiatric disorders is that overall functioning is generally not impaired. A person with delusional disorder may have impaired functioning in relation to their delusion and how it impacts their reality, but overall functioning is not significantly impaired. The delusions are also nonbizarre. As mentioned previously, when describing delusions as a symptom of other disorders, they are often quite unbelievable and bizarre. In contrast, in a delusional disorder, the belief is often a possible reality, and sometimes collateral information needs to be gathered to ensure the belief is in fact a delusion. This disorder also occurs more often in older patients. Many of the other disorders we have discussed present in early 20s to 30s. Delusional disorder, on the other hand, is common in people after the age of 40. Treatment for delusional disorder is a challenge. In many of the other psychotic disorders people at least acknowledge there is a problem because the disorder is distressing to them and causes a major impact in overall functioning. However, people with delusional disorder generally lack insight into the disorder or even a problem, making it difficult to treat. Antipsychotics should be offered as an initial treatment once the disorder is diagnosed as they have been effective in some cases. Unfortunately, they have been shown to have limited efficacy in the treatment of the disorder, but there seem to be no better pharmacologic options at this time. So a course of antipsychotics should be tried along with individual therapy.

Brief Psychotic Disorder

This is a rarer diagnosis than schizophrenia or schizoaffective disorder. It is classified by one or more psychotic symptoms (delusions, hallucinations, disorganized speech, or disorganized behavior) that last from one day to one month. About one quarter to one half of people with this diagnosis may go on to be diagnosed with schizophrenia or a mood disorder. The rest will undergo a course of antipsychotic treatment; they may or may not require hospitalization and individual therapy and will then return to their previous level of functioning. While schizophrenia and schizoaffective disorder may require lifelong treatment with antipsychotics, a brief psychotic disorder generally requires a short course of antipsychotics that can be slowly tapered off once the psychotic episode has resolved. The brief psychotic episode is sometimes in response to a marked life stressor or after giving birth; however, it can also occur without a marked life stressor.

Nonpsychotic Disorders

Psychotic symptoms can be present in other psychiatric disorders, medical illnesses, and substance-induced illnesses, and depending on the circumstances, antipsychotic treatment may be indicated. There are also some psychiatric disorders without psychotic symptoms that antipsychotics have been found useful for. These nonpsychotic disorders and the indications for antipsychotics will be discussed in the following pages.

Major Depressive Disorder with Psychotic Features

Major depressive disorder is characterized by a constellation of depressive symptoms that occur for at least a two-week period of time. The person must be either depressed or have overall lack of interest or pleasure with four other of the following symptoms: unintentional weight loss, insomnia or hypersomnia, increased or decreased psychomotor activity, decreased energy, feelings of worthlessness or guilt, decreased concentration, or recurrent thoughts of death or suicidal thoughts. These symptoms must cause significant distress or functional impairment. Some people with major depressive disorder also develop psychotic features. The psychotic features seen in this disorder are usually delusions or hallucinations. They can either be mood congruent, meaning they will have negative delusions that further their depressive symptoms. Or they can be mood incongruent, meaning they would be more positive and contradicting the person's depressive symptoms. The psychotic features are more often mood congruent. While major depressive disorder can often be treated with just an antidepressant, if there are psychotic features an antipsychotic is indicated. Multiple studies have shown that the combination of an antidepressant and an antipsychotic is more effective than either treatment alone. It is agreed that the initial course of treatment should be with both classes of medications; what is not well understood is how long treatment should continue after the remission of symptoms, specifically treatment with an antipsychotic. This is an area needing further research before clear guidelines and recommendations can be made.

Bipolar Disorder

Bipolar disorder has two different classifications that are based on severity of disease, specifically of the mania symptoms. The bipolar disorders are known to be disorders of mood dysregulation. People with bipolar disorder have extreme highs (euphoria) and extreme lows (depression). However, in order to be diagnosed with bipolar I disorder, the more severe type, a person only needs to meet criteria for one full manic episode. A manic episode is classified by a period of abnormally and persistently elevated, expansive, or irritable mood and abnormally increased energy for at least one week. During that period of time one must also experience three to four of the following symptoms with the elevated mood: grandiosity, decreased need for sleep, more talkative than usual, racing thoughts, easily distracted, increase in goal-directed activity, or excessive risky behavior. These behaviors and symptoms must be notably different from the person's normal behavior, and they must cause significant impairment in important areas of daily functioning such as social or occupational. Lifetime prevalence of bipolar I disorder is thought to be around 1%; however, more recently, this is thought that bipolar spectrum disorders are much more prevalent than 1%. Like many of the other psychiatric illnesses, the onset of the illness is usually in young adulthood, generally before the age of 30. Bipolar I disorder has the highest genetic link known of all of the major psychiatric disorders.

In order to meet criteria for bipolar II disorder, a person must have two different types of mood episodes. One must meet criteria for a current or past major depressive episode (same criteria apply as mentioned previously for a major depressive episode) and criteria for a current or past hypomanic episode. The general difference between a hypomanic episode and a manic episode is the duration of the episode and the severity of the symptoms. The symptoms of a manic episode must be present for one week, and the symptoms of a hypomanic episode have to be present for at least four days. Again they must meet three to four of the same criteria as a manic episode and the behavior must be a noticeable change from a person's baseline. However, the episodes must not be severe enough to cause a marked impairment in a person's daily functioning. Also, if the symptoms have psychotic features, it is considered more severe, and it cannot be classified as a hypomanic episode but could qualify as a manic episode.

Antipsychotics are indicated in treatment for both of these disorders but in slightly different ways. For treatment of an acute manic episode, an antipsychotic is always indicated. By definition, the acute manic episode does not require psychotic features, but psychosis is seen in many acute manic episodes. An antipsychotic can be used alone or with a mood stabilizer during the acute manic phase until stabilization. The typical antipsychotics have long been found useful as the sole treatment during the acute manic phase. In the more recent years, however, the atypical antipsychotics have all been studied extensively in the same role and have been found efficacious and are approved as monotherapy in acute mania. Some of the atypical antipsychotics have been studied in the use of maintenance treatment of bipolar disorder, meaning they have been found to be efficacious and are approved for use in between mood states in order to help prevent relapse into either a depressive or manic episode. Currently there are five atypical antipsychotics that have been approved for use during the maintenance phase of bipolar disorder, including aripiprazole, ziprasidone, quetiapine, olanzapine, and risperidone. The atypical antipsychotics have been shown to have some mood stabilization properties along with their antipsychotic properties, which is likely why they are beneficial in helping to prevent relapse of mood states. The decision about whether to use an antipsychotic alone or an antipsychotic with a mood stabilizer must be made on a case-by-case basis. Some of the factors to consider when making that decision include the severity of psychotic features during manic episodes, frequency of relapse, and potential side effects. Many of the atypical antipsychotics cause metabolic effects, including weight gain and increased lipids and glucose, putting people at risk of other medical complications down the road. These side effects will be discussed in greater detail in a later chapter, but it is important to consider these factors when trying to make a decision about the best medication regimen for an individual.

The final area of bipolar disorder that antipsychotics may be indicated in is bipolar depression. This has been a notoriously difficult mood state to treat. Partly because the first-line treatment for depression is a selective serotonin reuptake inhibitor (SSRI), however, using an antidepressant to treat depression in someone with bipolar disorder increases the risk of inducing a hypomanic or manic episode. At this point there is not good research to suggest that the addition of an antidepressant to a mood stabilizer is beneficial for bipolar depression. And so this has been an area of interest for further research and development of new, more efficacious medications. Currently there are three atypical antipsychotics that have been studied, found efficacious, and approved for the treatment of bipolar depression. Olanzapine has been studied in combination with an SSRI, fluoxetine, for bipolar depression. It has been approved as a combination drug called Symbyax (fluoxetine and olanzapine). However, it is not used frequently as a combination medication limits flexibility with dosing, and olanzapine is one of the worst offenders for metabolic side effects. Quetiapine has also been approved for bipolar depression and has been approved for use by itself. The short-term studies showed quetiapine to be successful by itself. But in the long-term studies that showed it to be continually efficacious, it was not used as a monotherapy; it was used in combination with a mood stabilizer. This should be taken into consideration if choosing to use quetiapine in the treatment of bipolar depression. Lastly, lurasidone, one of the newest atypical antipsychotics, has been approved for monotherapy or adjunct therapy with a mood stabilizer for bipolar depression. Lurasidone seems to have a better side effect profile than some of the other atypical antipsychotics, making it a promising medication for the future. However, it is still a newer medication, and longer-term studies and follow-ups will need to be continued in order to determine more completely its efficacy and safety profile.

Autism Spectrum Disorder

Autism spectrum disorder is a disorder characterized by persistent deficits in social communication and social interaction across multiple contexts. People with autism spectrum disorder also show restricted, repetitive patterns of behavior, interests, or activities. These symptoms must be present early in the developmental period and must cause significant impairment in functioning. The disorder is exactly as it is titled, a spectrum, and the presentations can be quite varied by symptom and by level of impairment. The treatment for people with autism spectrum disorder must be individualized, especially since the presentation can be so varied; however, the American Academy of Child and Adolescent Psychiatry has developed practice parameters in order to guide clinicians in their approach to treatment. Parts of those parameters provide guidelines in how to approach medication use for autism spectrum disorder. The basis of the guidelines is that medication can and should be offered as therapy if there is a specific target symptom or comorbid condition. One of the more upsetting features of autism spectrum disorder is the behavioral outbursts, irritability, and impulsivity that can lead to harm to the patient or others. Antipsychotics have been found to be helpful for some of these symptoms. Risperidone and aripiprazole have been approved for the treatment of irritability associated with autism. The irritability is primarily characterized by physical aggression and severe tantrum behavior. Other atypical antipsychotics have been studied for improvement in overall functioning as well as irritability and aggression and have shown some improvement, but only risperidone and aripiprazole have actually been FDA-approved.

Substance-Induced Psychotic Disorder

When trying to categorize psychotic disorders, one of the things that must always be considered is whether substances may be complicating the presentation. In order to meet criteria for a substance-induced psychotic disorder, one must have either delusions or hallucinations that developed during or soon after substance intoxication or withdrawal. The symptoms are often brief and resolve shortly after the drug is cleared, but some substances cause symptoms that last much longer. The treatment depends on the substance used and the person's agitation. As has been discussed previously, antipsychotics have been shown to improve irritability and aggression and are used to help with acute agitation in psychotic patients. The initial form of treatment for nearly every substance-induced psychosis is a calm environment. Many patients then would benefit from either a benzodiazepine or antipsychotic. Particularly for psychosis that is stimulated by dopamine, like from amphetamines, an antipsychotic is indicated and effective. For psychosis caused by substances not secondary to an increase in dopamine, starting with a calm environment and an anxiolytic, like a benzodiazepine, should be utilized first. If there is no improvement seen with a calm environment and anxiolytic and the person remains psychotic and agitated, then an antipsychotic is indicated. In the case of substance-induced psychosis, the antipsychotic is only indicated until there is resolution of symptoms and then it can be discontinued. If the patient only suffers from a substance-induced psychosis and not an underlying psychotic disorder, then symptoms should resolve shortly after the substance is cleared from the system and the antipsychotic is no longer required in order to control psychosis.

Psychotic Disorder Secondary to a Medical Condition

Some general medical conditions or acute medical illnesses can cause psychosis. This would be considered a secondary psychotic disorder. It can be difficult to determine the difference between a primary psychotic disorder, such as schizophrenia, and a secondary psychotic disorder caused by a medical condition. One of the largest general differences between the two is that in primary psychotic disorders generally a person's cognitive abilities and consciousness remain intact, whereas in psychotic disorders due to a general medical condition there is often an alteration in a person's cognition and/or level of consciousness. Other common occurrences with psychosis secondary to a medical condition are focal neurological abnormalities, abnormal vital signs (blood pressure, heart rate, respiratory rate, temperature), if hallucinations are present they are often visual instead of auditory, and if it occurs at an older age without a known underlying psychotic disorder it is more likely to be caused by a general medical condition. One of the other aspects to consider when determining if the psychosis is primary or secondary is the time course of the symptoms; if they seem to parallel the course of the medical illness, then it is likely secondary.

There are many different medical illnesses that could cause a secondary psychotic disorder; some of them are acute illnesses and others are chronic diseases. A discussion of the various different illnesses and diseases that could lead to psychosis is in itself enough material for a book, so in this section we will briefly touch on a few of the more common illnesses that lead to psychotic symptoms and the role of antipsychotics in those illnesses.

Delirium is one of the most common medical causes for psychosis. Delirium, however, is not a specific disease or illness but a syndrome defined by a set of symptoms. It is an acute confusional state with a decline in a known baseline of cognitive functions and intermittent fluctuations of level of consciousness. Delirium has a wide variety of causes. Some of the major causes include illness, medication or substances, or withdrawal from medication or substances. While delirium can be caused by virtually any illness, there are characteristics that make a person more vulnerable, and there are certain illnesses that are more likely to cause delirium. Some risk factors to getting delirium include older age, preexisting brain damage, malnutrition, and sensory impairment. Any kind of illness can cause delirium; even illnesses that do not directly impact the brain can worsen, impact the rest of the body, and eventually cause imbalances that affect the brain. Some types of illnesses are more likely than others to cause delirium and include infections, electrolyte abnormalities, liver disease, and endocrine disease. While delirium does not have to include symptoms of psychosis, it often does. The treatment for delirium is based around identification of the underlying cause and treatment of that underlying condition. If there are psychotic symptoms or agitation during states of confusion, antipsychotics are indicated for symptom management. However, there are no psychotropics that are FDA-approved for the treatment of delirium at this time. There is a lack of randomized controlled trials to guide pharmacologic treatment at this time; however, haloperidol has become the standard agent used despite the lack of FDA approval. One of the main reasons is that it has few anticholinergic effects, which could worsen underlying conditions. Other atypical antipsychotics that are used for the treatment of psychosis or agitation in delirium are risperidone, olanzapine, and quetiapine. These medications should be used while a person is delirious in order to control the symptoms. Once the underlying cause of the delirium is treated, the psychosis and agitation should have resolved, and the antipsychotics can be weaned off and do not need to be continued.

While nearly any disease can lead to delirium, which often includes some type of psychotic features, there are other illnesses that are more likely to cause a secondary psychosis which can be broken down into category of illnesses. Diseases of the endocrine system are systemic illnesses that often affect the brain and lead to a secondary psychosis. Most notably, thyroid disease, either hypo- or hyperthyroidism, if untreated can present with psychotic symptoms. Other endocrine diseases that lead to secondary psychosis include endocrine tumors that produce another substance such as steroid-producing tumors or insulin-producing tumors. Autoimmune diseases are another category of illness that can lead to secondary psychosis. Lupus is probably the most common offender in this category and actually so often can cause psychosis that psychotic symptoms are actually part of the diagnostic criteria for the disease. There are multiple infections that impact the brain and can lead to psychosis, including malaria and toxoplasmosis. Two infections that can cause psychotic symptoms if untreated are HIV and neurosyphilis, both of which are treatable diseases that affect the brain and can cause psychotic symptoms.

In all situations of secondary psychosis if the psychotic symptoms are distressing or dangerous to the person or people around them, they should be treated with an antipsychotic. However, the medication is merely serving the purpose of symptom regulation, and the ultimate treatment goal is the primary source of illness. If for example, the thyroid disease is properly treated, then the psychotic symptoms will also remit, and there will be no need for long-term treatment with antipsychotics.

The previous pages explore a variety of areas of disease and illness, either primarily psychotic or secondarily psychotic where antipsychotics are indicated for use. As with most medications, when speaking about them broadly, one can assume that the targeted patient is a young to middle-aged adult. As with all medications, when deciding whether or not to use them, you must take into consideration what other health problems a person has. But even with otherwise healthy individuals, there are some special groups that require a different kind of consideration when determining application and use of antipsychotics, including the elderly, children, and pregnant women. The use of antipsychotics in these special groups will be discussed in the next few pages.

ANTIPSYCHOTIC USE IN SPECIAL GROUPS

The Elderly

Elderly patients pose a variety of potential problems when considering prescribing any psychiatric medication, and antipsychotics are no different. The geriatric patient in general is considered more at risk to experience side effects of medications and will often experience side effects and efficacy at doses lower than needed in a younger adult. But at the same time, the mental illnesses that affect the young adult and middle-aged adult often continue to cause distress to the older adult along with a new set of distressing neurocognitive disorders. The situation is often complicated by other medical illnesses that the geriatric patient has and often takes medication for. So the risks and benefits of disease and treatment must be carefully considered when determining whether to treat with an antipsychotic. Because it is often unclear what a therapeutic dose will be, especially for an elderly patient, and the situation is complicated by all of the previously mentioned factors, the saying "start low and go slow" has become a commonly used phrase to guide initiation of a psychotropic medication for a geriatric patient. Meaning, start the patient at the lowest dose possible and very slowly increase the dose while monitoring for a response in symptoms and watching for the development of side effects. The use of antipsychotics in specific disorders of the elderly will be discussed in further detail.

Schizophrenia

There is a belief that as patients with schizophrenia age, they may require lower dosages than when they were younger or just compared with younger patients in general. Once someone with schizophrenia who has been maintained on antipsychotics grows beyond the age of 60, it is standard practice to at least attempt to gradually decrease their medication dose to see if they could be maintained at a lower dose. The elderly population may be more susceptible to side effects like dystonias or Parkinsonian movements. Because of this, the atypical antipsychotics may be more desirable in this population. However, these come with their own potential side effects like orthostatic hypotension and anticholinergic effects, which can be more dangerous in the elderly population. Another complicating factor when considering antipsychotic use in the elderly is that the use of atypical antipsychotics in elderly patients with dementia has been associated with an increased risk of death. Currently there is a black box warning on all atypical antipsychotics that indicates a higher risk of mortality when used in treating elderly patients with dementia. The reason for the increased mortality is not well understood, making it difficult to use this information when trying to decide on a medication to use for psychotic disorders in the elderly. The black box warning has not been applied to the typical antipsychotics, but it is not clearly understood why the risk would be higher with the atypicals, complicating the decision to use antipsychotics. Overall, generally the risks of untreated schizophrenia outweigh the risks of antipsychotic use; however, as the risk of antipsychotic use in the elderly is high, the decision to use them and the dosing should be carefully considered.

Agitation and Psychosis

Many elderly patients with chronic dementia or a decompensated medical illness will suffer with agitation and/or psychotic symptoms. These symptoms will sometimes be improved with treatment of the disease, but, for example, with dementia there is a chronic and poorly responsive course. The agitated and psychotic symptoms are not only distressing to caregivers, but they also can be dangerous to the person suffering from them. The options for treatment are somewhat limited, and antipsychotics have been used for years even though they have a less than ideal side effect profile for the elderly and especially for the elderly with dementia. The same concerns that were discussed earlier when using antipsychotics in the elderly with schizophrenia also apply to their use for agitation and psychosis in other illnesses. The first approach to a patient with dementia who is agitated or has psychotic symptoms would be to treat any complicating medical illnesses and work to reorient the patient. If the person continues to be psychotic or agitated and is not responding to other more benign medications, then an atypical antipsychotic could be used and can be beneficial. Generally, the typical antipsychotics are avoided for the treatment of agitation in the elderly because of the increased risk of movement side effects.

Bipolar Disorder

Unlike schizophrenia, bipolar disorder is known to worsen with age as well as the overall dysfunction that often comes with the disorder. Not everyone with bipolar disorder will be taking an antipsychotic; however, some will be maintained on one. It is also known that if a person is well managed on a treatment and then stops and has a mood episode, he or she may not respond to that treatment again. There is currently not enough research on the use of antipsychotics in the elderly with bipolar disorder to give clear guidance on usage. Therefore, each person's situation must be considered individually, weighing the risks of the side effects of antipsychotics in the elderly, as mentioned previously, versus the risks of stopping an antipsychotic and inducing a mood episode.

In general when considering an antipsychotic in the elderly, it is important to keep in mind the other medical risk factors they have and the increased risk of side effects. Each case should be considered individually, and more research is necessary to help guide clinical practice. Currently general practice is to proceed with caution with an understanding that there can be a time and situation to use antipsychotics in the elderly.

Children

Overall, there is less use of psychiatric medications and especially antipsychotics in children. There is a lack of data on the long-term consequences of drug therapy in childhood for many areas of functioning in adulthood. Another reason for a decreased use of antipsychotics in childhood is that the majority of illnesses in which an antipsychotic would be indicated are not prevalent until late adolescence or early adulthood. That being said, antipsychotics are used in childhood illnesses at times, and there are certain things to consider when using them with the pediatric population. In studies that have been done thus far, there does not seem to be evidence that children are any less tolerant of these medications than adults. However, similarly to the geriatric population, children require lower doses of antipsychotics than their adult counterpart. In childhood schizophrenia and bipolar disorder, the use of antipsychotics has been found to be beneficial, and the choice of antipsychotic is often made based on the side effect profile. As the typical antipsychotics have the potential side effect of a nonreversible movement disorder, tardive dyskinesia, and these children will likely be taking an antipsychotic for years, it is common to try an atypical antipsychotic first. The most troublesome side effect of the atypicals for the pediatric population is the risk of metabolic changes, but some are more likely to cause changes than others, which should be considered when choosing an agent.

While antipsychotics seem to have a role in childhood schizophrenia and bipolar disorder, their use in children with developmental disorders like autism has a more clearly defined role. In fact, risperidone was the first drug approved by the FDA for the treatment of some behavioral aspects of autism. Along that same line, antipsychotics have been used to control behavior of children who have a behavioral disorder without a developmental disorder. This has not been well validated, yet is still often used. This use could be paralleled with using antipsychotics to treat agitated elderly patients. It is most commonly used this way in the inpatient setting when the child's behaviors are not only distressing but are also dangerous to the child and to others.

In general, antipsychotics have some role in childhood treatment; however, it is still not clearly defined. The use of antipsychotics to treat behavioral disorders in a child with developmental disorders has been validated, they seem to be helpful in psychotic disorders like schizophrenia and bipolar disorder, and their use in treating behaviors not associated with a developmental disorder is not validated. When determining whether or not to treat with an antipsychotic, for the pediatric patient one of the most important aspects in the decision-making process is involving the parents, as they are the primary decision makers for the minor. Again, it becomes a risk versus benefit scenario where it would be important to consider the risk to the child's development and risk of side effects versus the benefit the child would receive from a better managed mental illness.

Pregnant Women

The last few pages have discussed the use of antipsychotics in the special populations of the elderly and children. The take-home message has been that there is some role for antipsychotics, and it will always be a difficult decision to make because of the risk that goes along with their use. The population of pregnant women may be the most difficult population to make treating decisions for because you are no longer worried just about how the medication might have an impact on the person with the mental illness, but how the medication might affect their pregnancy or how discontinuing treatment might affect their pregnancy. This is at the core of making all treatment decisions with pregnant women, and antipsychotics are no outlier. This dilemma is not one limited to psychotropics, so the FDA has created categories to indicate the level of risk potential for a medication to cause fetal injury. There are five categories that are complex and will not be discussed in detail here; however, antipsychotics fall into only two of these categories, so they will be explained. There are two scenarios that may occur in pregnancy to indicate use of an antipsychotic.

First, if a woman is already maintained on an antipsychotic and then becomes pregnant or is trying to become pregnant, the question arises about whether or not to stop the medication. In that instance, it is important to compare the risk of the specific medication she is taking with the risk of her mental illness. This depends on the individual. If the woman is diagnosed with schizophrenia and is functioning well on her antipsychotic and it is known that the last time she stopped, she quickly became psychotic and dangerous and was hospitalized, then it is clear that she and her fetus likely benefit more from staying on the antipsychotic. Unfortunately, not all cases are this clear.

The second scenario is with a woman who is pregnant and becomes psychotic or has a first occurrence of bipolar disorder during pregnancy. In this case again, one needs to consider how severe the presentation of the illness is and if there are other, potentially less harmful, medications that could be used. If the illness is severe and there is concern for the woman's ability to care for herself or cause harm and no less harmful medications are available, then it is generally considered appropriate to provide treatment with an antipsychotic.

All of the antipsychotics cross the placenta to some degree, and there is some risk of congenital malformations. However, there is no known proven relationship between the antipsychotics and specific birth defects. Nearly all of the antipsychotics are categorized with a class C pregnancy risk. This means that risk has not been ruled out but that there have not been adequate human studies. There have been animal reproduction studies that show an adverse effect on the fetus, but without adequate human studies, potential benefits may outweigh the risks. One of the antipsychotics, clozapine, has a classification of category B. This means either that animal studies have not shown a risk and there are no adequate human studies, or that animal studies have shown a risk but there are also adequate human studies that have failed to demonstrate a risk to the fetus at any trimester. This does not mean that if a pregnant woman is on an antipsychotic, she should be switched to clozapine, as it has many of its own side effects to consider; however, if a woman is already maintained on clozapine and becomes pregnant, it makes it more likely that she should simply stay on the medication throughout the pregnancy.

For use in all of the special populations, the take-home point is that each must be considered on an individual basis. In the elderly population, they likely need lower doses and are at more risk for side effects. In the pediatric population, they will need lower doses, and there is the potential for blunting cognitive development. Finally, in the pregnant population, one must consider not only the effects on the patient but on the fetus as well. There is a role for antipsychotics in all of these groups and scenarios; they just need to be considered as a special population.

Chapter 6

Risks, Misuse, and Overdose

The prescription and accessibility of medications carry significant risks and dangers. The goal of any drug, after all, is to alleviate a problem by changing the body's biology and chemistry. It would be naive to think that a person's physiology could be changed by a drug in only the intended ways. Any drug, including seemingly harmless medications, like aspirin and Tylenol, can have unforeseen consequences. Adverse effects of medications are the norm, not the exception, across all fields of medicine. Medication will only be beneficial when the problems addressed by the medications are greater than the problems created. The risks of medications are serious when the medications are taken correctly, but when medications are used incorrectly, the problems are exponentially worse. Medications are used incorrectly for a variety of reasons. They could be abused as street drugs, used in excess as a suicide attempt, or accidently misused by a well-meaning patient. The risks involved with antipsychotics are complicated by the nature of the illnesses they treat. Patients are less likely to be organized, less likely to have access to support in the community, and may be more likely to attempt to hurt themselves. Therefore, responsible psychiatrists are well-aware of the myriad side effects of antipsychotics and the consequences of misuse and overdose.

SIDE EFFECTS

There are many concerns involved with antipsychotic medications. As a class of drugs, antipsychotics have several side effects that make them unappealing or intolerable. As discussed elsewhere in this text, antipsychotics can generally be divided into typical (first-generation) antipsychotics and atypical (second-generation) antipsychotics. While many of the potential side effects can occur with any antipsychotic, there are clear patterns and distinctions between these two major classes of antipsychotics.

Biologic Basis of the Movement Disorders

One of the most concerning groups of side effects associated with antipsychotics involves movement. The principal reason behind this phenomenon is that antipsychotics block dopamine, which is the neurotransmitter that mediates movement.

The typical antipsychotics, which include haloperidol (Haldol), fluphenazine (Prolixin), perphenazine (Trilafon), and chlorpromazine (Thorazine), are commonly associated with movement disorders called extrapyramidal symptoms (EPS). The name of these disorders derives from the neuroanatomy of movement. Voluntary movement involves tracts of neurons in the brain and spinal cord that are collectively referred to as the pyramidal system. These tracts originate in the part of the brain's cortex responsible for motor (motor and premotor cortex) and are organized in the medulla, the lower portion of the brain stem. They proceed through specific tracts in the spinal cord and connect with muscles through the body. When someone wants to raise his or her hand in class, the brain sends signals through the pyramidal system that activates the appropriate muscles that facilitates the desired motion. There is a parallel neural pathway called the extrapyramidal system (outside the pyramidal system) that is responsible for involuntary movement and coordination. The extrapyramidal system has origins in the part of the brain's cortex responsible for sensory perception (sensory cortex) and the basal ganglia, a deep brain system that regulates the coordination of movement. The neurons of the extrapyramidal system travel through the brain stem's pons and medulla and then through different tracts in the spinal cord and connect to muscles throughout the body. The movements involved in the side effects collectively called EPS are involuntary, poorly coordinated movements that result from a dysfunctional extrapyramidal system. As noted previously, the principal reason antipsychotics interfere with movement relates to the mechanism of action of the drug. Antipsychotics block dopamine, which is one of the neurotransmitters that are responsible for movement. Therefore, if dopamine is blocked, movement will be affected.

Types of Movement Disorders

Acute Movement Disorders

The EPS can be differentiated by symptoms and time course. Acute symptoms begin within minutes, hours, or days of initiating treatment. Acute forms of EPS include neuroleptic-induced Parkinsonism, akathisia, and acute dystonia.

Neuroleptic-Induced Parkinsonism

As the name implies, neuroleptic-induced Parkinsonism describes symptoms that are similar to Parkinson's disease. Parkinson's disease is a movement disorder that is characterized by rigidity, shuffling gait, and a specific tremor. However, the cause of symptoms differs. Parkinson's disease is caused by degeneration of dopaminergic cells that begin in the substantia nigra, an area of the brain associated with the basal ganglia, which is responsible for the coordination of movement. The degeneration of these cells often occurs spontaneously, and researchers have not discovered exact causes. In some cases, brain trauma or certain pesticides are believed to trigger Parkinson's. The degeneration of dopaminergic cells essentially leads to a decrease of dopamine produced in the substantia nigra. Neuroleptic-induced Parkinsonism is caused by a blockade of dopamine in other parts of the brain, after it was synthesized in the substantia nigra and distributed throughout the brain appropriately. However, in both cases the end results is a dysfunctional dopamine system, which results in similar symptoms.

There are five major pathways that connect the basal ganglia to other parts of the brain: motor, oculomotor, associative, limbic, and orbitofrontal. As discussed, dopamine is the predominant neurotransmitter that travels along these routes. While decreased levels of dopamine lead to dysfunction in all pathways in Parkinson's disease, neuroleptic-induced Parkinsonism typically involves the motor pathway. The major symptoms are tremor, rigidity, bradykinesia (slow movement), and postural instability.

Tremor, or involuntary shaking of hands, is perhaps the most recognizable symptom of Parkinsonism. There are many types of tremors, and they are differentiated by when they are most active and their speed. Intention tremors are most active when a patient uses his or her hands for a specific purpose. For example, a patient may be fine at rest, but when he or she reaches over for a glass of water, his or her hand may visibly shake. Resting tremors work in the opposite direction. If a patient had a resting tremor, the hand would shake in a resting position, but the tremor would disappear when he or she reached for the glass of water and took a drink. The speed of a tremor, called the frequency, is expressed in hertz, cycles per second. A tremor with a frequency of 10 hertz means the hand goes up and down 10 times per second, which would be a relatively fast tremor. A slow tremor would have a frequency of 2 or 3 hertz. Parkinsonism is associated with a resting tremor of 4–6 hertz. The tremor that is produced by Parkinsonism is known as a "pill-rolling" tremor. This refers to early techniques of manufacturing pills, whereby a pharmacist would roll the pills by rubbing his or her thumb and index finger in a circular motion. Patients with Parkinsonism involuntarily mimic this motion at rest.

Patients with Parkinsonism are often rigid. This results from abnormal levels of contraction in certain muscle groups. Doctors refer to two types of rigidity commonly seen in Parkinsonism. Lead-pipe rigidity is when muscle groups have a consistently high muscle tone. If one were to move the arms of an affected patient, it would be very difficult, as if he or she were willfully resisting. Cogwheel rigidity results from an inconsistent level of muscle tone. A frequent test for cogwheel rigidity involves the doctor holding the patient's hand or wrist and moving the forearm in a circular motion while keeping the elbow steady. The patient is asked to relax his or her arm. Normally, the forearm should move smoothly. However, if the patient has cogwheel rigidity, the arm will seem to get stuck or caught up several times in the course of making the circle.

Other classic signs of Parkinsonism are bradykinesia (slow movement) and shuffling gait. The entire process of planning, initiating, and executing movement is delayed. When patients do move, they often take small steps, barely clearing the ground, and walk hunched over. These movement difficulties lead to significant impairment in accomplishing everyday tasks.

Postural instability refers to Parkinson's patients' difficulty maintaining a sturdy balance. Balance is a difficult achievement that healthy people take for granted every day. However, in order to stay upright, the brain must have an instantaneous and accurate knowledge of where all parts of the body are, a process known as proprioception, and the flexibility to make rapid minor adjustments when there is a chance of taking a tumble. For example, when healthy individuals walk down a street, the path is rarely perfectly smooth, and not all obstacles are foreseen. When there is an unexpected branch on the ground or a crack in the sidewalk, the brain instantly sends signals to the muscles to move the body in perfectly accurate positions to stay right side up. Falls in the healthy population are very unusual, occurring several times per year, if that, unless someone decides to take up skateboarding or ice-skating. Otherwise, the brain's ability to always know whether the limbs are in space and make rapid, flexible adjustments is impressively consistent. This flexibility is lacking in Parkinson's patients and leads to frequent falls. Affected individuals cannot react quickly when knocked even slightly off-balance, leading to falls that can cause serious injuries, including broken bones and head trauma. Furthermore, even when a healthy person does fall, for example when skiing or hiking in icy conditions, he or she is still able to make fast movements to mitigate the damage of the fall. People are almost always able to throw a hand out to soften the blow, sometimes leading to broken wrists, but preventing trauma to the face or brain. This is not the case with a Parkinsonian fall. Patients may not be able to soften the blow, and an innocent trip over some clothes could lead to a trip to the emergency room.

When these symptoms and signs are associated with Parkinson's disease, they are expected to worsen over time. There are medications and interventions for Parkinson's disease, but there are no cures. Neuroleptic-induced Parkinsonism, however, is more readily addressed. As mentioned previously, high doses or typical antipsychotics are most likely to cause neuroleptic-induced Parkinsonism. Therefore, decreasing the dose of antipsychotics and/or switching to an atypical antipsychotic, like quetiapine, risperidone, or clozapine, may alleviate symptoms. As with other EPS, adding anticholinergic medications like Benadryl or benztropine decreases symptoms as well.

Acute Dystonia

Acute dystonia refers to the sudden contraction of a muscle or muscle group. The mechanism of these contractions is that dopamine facilitates the ability to release muscles and move normally. Without dopamine, muscles get "locked" and patients are unable to move them. This side effect is very painful and scary for patients.

The nature of the acute dystonia depends on which muscle contracts. One common acute dystonia is called torticollis. Torticollis is a contraction of the sternocleidomastoid muscle in the neck, which connects parts of the skull to the collar bone. Rolling the neck in circles is dependent on the sternocleidomastoid muscle. Someone with torticollis will have his or her head pointed down and to the side. Another form of acute dystonia is called oculogyric crisis, which involves a contraction of the muscles around the eyes and will result in an affected patient's eyes fixed in a given location or rotating uncontrollably. If laryngeal muscles (small muscles around the voice box) are affected during an acute dystonia, breathing can be affected. Although acute dystonias are very painful, they are rarely dangerous. However, if laryngeal muscles are involved, patients can stop breathing. However, that is an exceedingly rare occurrence.

Acute dystonias as a whole are very rare reactions and typically occur when large doses of typical agents are administered to patients who are naive to antipsychotics (have never been exposed to them before). Acute dystonias are also more likely to occur when antipsychotics are given intramuscularly instead of orally because they enter the bloodstream and exert effects much more quickly. Therefore, an agitated, young patient who is experiencing a first-break psychotic episode is at particular risk of developing an acute dystonic reaction because he or she will likely require intramuscular medication. Intramuscular injections work faster and can sedate patients quicker than oral medications. Therefore, if the medical staff is more concerned about safety, the patient will be more likely to receive an intramuscular injection. Male patients are therefore more likely to experience acute dystonias than female patients because they generally raise more concerns about violence and are more likely to receive injections. Younger patients experiencing a first break will also by definition be naive to antipsychotics. The treatment is an intramuscular anticholinergic medication, like diphenhydramine (Benadryl) or benztropine (Cogentin). The reasons these medications work involve a complicated neural connection involving the dopamine and acetylcholine pathways in the brain.

Akathisia

A common EPS is akathisia. Although listed here under acute movement disorders, akathisias can be acute or emerge over the course of weeks. Akathisia is an uncomfortable, tingling sensation involving the legs. An affected patient may feel the need to walk around and be unable to sit still. Akathisia is similar to restless leg syndrome (RLS), but it occurs at all times in the day instead of exclusively at night. The sensation is similar to feeling like legs are "asleep." Patients describe feeling uncomfortable as rest and physically agitated. Akathisia is difficult to identify and treat for several reasons. First, it is difficult for patients to describe, especially if they are psychotic and have difficulty expressing even simple ideas. It is also difficult to diagnose based on a patient's behavior. A person suffering from akathisia may be noted to pace around the units of a hospital. However, psychotic and agitated patients will also pace around units. Therefore, it is difficult for psychiatrists to decide what to do when they see their patients furiously pacing. Do they need more antipsychotics to calm down or less antipsychotics to decrease the akathisias? Treatment for akathisias includes a decreased dose of antipsychotics or a switch from typical to atypical antipsychotics because atypicals in general are less likely to cause EPS. There are also medications that can relieve akathisias, including anticholinergic medication (Benadryl or benztropine), benzodiazepines (antianxiety medications), or propranolol (a blood pressure medication). Akathisas are a major reason why patients stop taking antipsychotics. Therefore, when patients complain of symptoms, it is important that psychiatrists take this seriously, even if akathisia is not life-threatening and does not lead to more serious medical complications.

Tardive Dyskinesia

As opposed to the other movement disorders, which occur after minutes, days, or weeks of initiating antipsychotics, tardive dyskinesia often takes years to develop. The term "dyskinesia" implies a movement disorder, and the term "tardive" means late-occurring. Tardive dyskinesia is a condition that emerges long after an antipsychotic medication is initiated and can last long after the medication is withdrawn.

Patients with tardive dyskinesia have rhythmic, tremor-like movements of different body parts. Often the face is involved and can manifest in tongue movements, as if the patient is constantly chewing or rolling over the tongue. Sucking or lip-smacking movements are often seen. Patients can appear as if they are grimacing. Other common manifestations of tardive dyskinesia involve the upper body. It may look like a patient is constantly rocking or gyrating his or her body above the waist. The chances of developing tardive dyskinesia are a function of the amount of antipsychotics a patient has taken and the length of treatment. Therefore, tardive dyskinesia is most commonly seen in chronically hospitalized elderly patients with psychotic illnesses, like schizophrenia, that do not respond to normal doses of antipsychotics. These patients generally require high doses of antipsychotics and have likely taken them for many decades. Since they are elderly and schizophrenia usually emerges in young adulthood, most, if not all, of their antipsychotics have been typical antipsychotics. Atypicals, which have a decreased risk of EPS, only gained widespread popularity in the 1990s. Today's elderly patients with schizophrenia likely began taking medications around the 1960s. Even though atypical antipsychotics have been used extensively for over 20 years, psychiatrists avoid changing medications if patients are psychiatrically stable. Therefore, many of these elderly patients have taken relatively high-dose typical antipsychotics for over 50 years. These patients are extremely likely to suffer from some form of tardive dyskinesia. Indeed, studies have shown rates of tardive dyskinesia to be as high as 60% in the elderly, hospitalized population.

The neurological mechanism of tardive dyskinesia is complicated and is the subject of significant amounts of research. The most current explanations are counterintuitive. Tardive dyskinesia is caused by antipsychotics that block dopamine in the brain. However, as a response, the brain increases the dopamine receptors on neurons because it senses that something is wrong, a process known as upregulation. Therefore, over time, antipsychotics lead to the proliferation of dopamine receptors in the brain that cause certain pathways to show increased levels of dopaminergic activity. This increased activity in the motor pathways of the brain leads to the extra movements seen in tardive dyskinesia. Therefore, one way to precipitate tardive dyskinesia is to stop taking antipsychotics after many years. If an elderly patient who has been compliant with medications for a long period of time, the brain would have upregulated dopamine receptors in the brain as a response. After antipsychotics are stopped abruptly and dopamine is no longer blocked in any capacity, there is a flurry of activity along the dopaminergic pathways, leading to the involuntary rocking motions of tardive dyskinesia.

As a result of the cause of the condition, the treatment, oddly enough, is higher doses of antipsychotics. The most reasonable reaction to developing a side effect of a medication is to stop taking it, but in this case, it is not an effective measure, let alone the implications for a patient's psychiatric condition. The drugs that caused the condition can address it, by blocking dopamine transmission at the upregulated receptors. As mentioned earlier, typical antipsychotics are more likely to cause all EPS, including tardive dyskinesia, so a common treatment strategy is to switch patients from typical to atypical agents. Clozapine, specifically, has been associated with the lowest incidence of tardive dyskinesia. Vitamin E was also thought to treat tardive dyskinesia but has lost favor among practitioners due to limited results.

The unfortunate reality is that there is no treatment for tardive dyskinesia, which causes elderly patients significant embarrassment and inability to accomplish everyday tasks. Because the side effect does not generally occur for decades, many doctors avoid discussing it with their patients. After all, the doctor will most likely be long gone by the time the patient develops symptoms. However, for a patient to make a fully informed decision about whether to take antipsychotics, he or she must be made aware of all the possible side effects, to a reasonable degree. In fact, several successful lawsuits have been brought against psychiatrists many years after they did not think to disclose the risks of tardive dyskinesia to young patients.

Practice guidelines require psychiatrists to objectively assess involuntary movements for all patients who are prescribed antipsychotics on an annual basis. The assessment, which takes between 5 and 10 minutes, is called the Abnormal Involuntary Movement Scale (AIMS). Psychiatrists essentially ask patients if they have noticed involuntary movements and then observe patients in several positions and assess the degree of the movements.

Sedation

Antipsychotics cause varying degrees of sedation or tiredness. Sometimes, this is not necessarily a side effect but rather an intended effect of the medication. For example, if patients are agitated or aggressive, psychiatrists often prescribe medications with the intent of making patients sedated so they will be less likely to hurt themselves and others. Furthermore, patients with acute psychotic symptoms often have poor sleep, so giving sedating antipsychotics at night relieves this symptom in addition to the broader psychotic illness.

However, sedation is often an unwelcome and unpleasant side effect of antipsychotics. The low-potency typical antipsychotics, including chlorpromazine, are significantly sedating. Also, atypical agents like clozapine, olanzapine, and quetiapine cause significant sedation. Clozapine is the antipsychotic linked with the highest rates of sedation. Sedation is a major reason why patients stop taking antipsychotics. It can make working or accomplishing basic activities very difficult. To illustrate this, in psychiatric hospitals, there are many groups, including education, art, and dance, offered throughout the day. In each of these groups, it is almost given that several patients will be asleep in their chair due to the sedating effects of antipsychotics.

There are several strategies psychiatrists can take to minimize sedation as an adverse effect. If sedation is a problem, psychiatrists can lower the dose or switch to a less-sedating agent, including haloperidol, aripiprazole, ziprasidone, or risperidone. Another common strategy is to give all the medication before bedtime, when patients do not mind feeling sedated. Patients can also take activating medications to counteract sedation, including stimulants, typically given to patients with attention-deficit hyperactivity disorder (ADHD). Lastly, patients can use a timeless remedy used by billions of people worldwide daily to provide a jump start: coffee.

Metabolic Syndrome and Cardiovascular Risk

Currently, atypical antipsychotics, like risperidone (Risperdal), quetiapine (Seroquel), aripiprazole (Abilify), and clozapine (Clozaril), are used more than typicals, because they have fewer EPS. Also, as discussed elsewhere in this text, atypical antipsychotics are more effective in decreasing the negative symptoms of schizophrenia. The major side effect associated with atypical antipsychotics is metabolic syndrome.

Metabolism refers to the process by which the body uses food to fuel the biochemical process that facilitates normal physiology and functioning. Metabolic syndrome is, as the name implies, a disorder involving how the body metabolizes (breaks down) those calories. Metabolic syndrome is diagnosed with the presence of three or more of the following five medical conditions:

- Abdominal (central) obesity. Having a large waist or an "apple" shaped body. It is counterintuitive, but fat, or adipose tissue, affects the body differently depending on where it accumulates. Fat located in the abdominal area is worse for metabolism and cardiovascular health than fat located in other parts of the body, including hips, thighs, or bust. It is very difficult for medical organizations to agree on a specific waist circumference that constitutes abdominal obesity. It largely depends on gender, ethnicity, and body frame. However, when patients have a body mass index (BMI) greater than 30 kg/m^2, abdominal obesity can be assumed.

- Elevated blood pressure. Systolic blood pressure greater than 130 or diastolic blood pressure greater than 85, or, if a patient has received treatment for hypertension.

- Elevated glucose (high blood sugar). This can be tested several ways. Generally, clinicians test fasting blood glucose (glucose in the blood when the patient has not eaten for at least six hours). An elevated value would be greater than 100 mg/dl or if the patient has ever been diagnosed with type II diabetes mellitus.

- High serum triglycerides. Triglycerides are one type of "bad" cholesterol and are essentially fat found floating around in the blood. Increased triglycerides are generally considered to be greater than 150 mg/dl or if the patient is being treated for this condition.

- Low high-density lipoprotein (HDL) levels. HDL is the "good" cholesterol and having lower values is a risk factor for cardiovascular disease. Low HDL is generally considered to be less than 40 mg/dl in males and 50 mg/dl in females or if the patient is being treated with medication to address this specific lipid condition.

Antipsychotics, especially atypical antipsychotics, increase the risk of metabolic syndrome, which is dangerous for many reasons. It increases the risk of diabetes and cardiovascular events, including heart attacks and strokes. The exact mechanism behind the heart attacks and strokes is complicated. Essentially elevated cholesterol and blood glucose levels increase the risks of damage, inflammation, and plaques that build up in blood vessels. These vessels supply the heart tissue with oxygen-rich blood and also serve as the exit route for newly oxygenated blood from the lungs to be pumped by the heart throughout the entire body. The most import organ that needs the oxygen-rich blood is the brain, which is the second recipient of the blood, after the heart itself. The heart provides itself with blood with the coronary arteries and then sends blood directly up to the brain through the carotid arteries. When there is enough inflammation and fatty build in the vessels, the plaque can become unstable, break off the vessel wall, and cause a block further down the blood vessel. When this happens in the coronary artery system, it leads to a heart attack or myocardial infarction. When it happens in the carotid arteries, it leads to a cerebrovascular accident, also known as a CVA, or a stroke. One study found that 32% of patients with chronic schizophrenia have metabolic syndrome.

There are several ways to address metabolic syndrome in patients taking antipsychotics. The first step is prevention and early detection. Before initiating antipsychotics, physicians should establish patients' baseline weight, BMI, blood pressure, cholesterol level, and blood sugar level. All of these measures should be taken every three months to identify if patients' metabolism is being significantly adversely affected by antipsychotics. Physicians should also educate their patients about metabolic syndrome and encourage them to eat and exercise accordingly. Patients should be on low-calorie, low-fat, and low-sugar diets. Patients should also exercise as much as possible, within reason. The association of metabolic syndrome and antipsychotics is especially relevant given the increasing rates of obesity in the general population. The prevalence of metabolic syndrome in patients who take antipsychotics is between 25% and 50%, depending on the study.

As mental health practitioners know too well, it is very difficult to change psychiatric patients' lifestyle habits to prevent or reverse metabolic syndrome. To be fair, it is very difficult for even a general primary care physician to motivate a patient without a mental illness to eat healthier food and exercise more. As people age, they get more stuck into patterns that become second nature. Food, especially relatively inexpensive, high-fat, high-carbohydrate options like fast food, is a comfort item. It is very difficult to convince someone to exchange the burger and fries for a spinach salad with walnuts and grilled salmon, when the latter option is twice as expensive and takes three times as long to prepare. Exercise as well is time-consuming and painful at times. It also can be expensive if a patient needs to join a gym or buy equipment and clothing.

These are the challenges faced by every patient in the country who needs to improve their lifestyle. To be successful, patients must be motivated, focused, self-confident, and often supported by friends or family. This is why patients with serious mental illnesses, like schizophrenia, have such a difficult time changing their lifestyle and, ultimately, die on average 10 to 20 years earlier than people without serious mental illnesses. Lack of motivation is one of the classic negative symptoms of schizophrenia, making it very difficult to organize and put effort into self-care. Also, patients with serious mental illnesses often have a diminished self-esteem, so they are less likely to invest time and energy into their own well-being. Further, patients with serious mental illnesses are less likely to be part of a community of people who cheer them on and cook them healthy food. This is yet another reason that the strength of the psychiatrist-patient relationship is critical. If the patient has trust and faith in the psychiatrist, he or she is more likely to follow the doctor's advice. If the psychiatrist simply directs a patient to change his or her life in a preachy and condescending way, he or she is unlikely to foster any meaningful change. The psychiatrist has the best chance helping patients take steps if he or she takes the time to work with the patient, understands his or her difficulties, empathizes with the challenges in overcoming hurdles, sets realistic goals, and cheers on any positive changes, no matter how big or small.

If a patient is diagnosed with metabolic syndrome despite his/her best attempts at eating well and exercising, the antipsychotic medication should be adjusted. Within the class of atypical antipsychotics, certain medications are more likely than others to cause metabolic syndrome. Olanzapine has been shown to cause the highest rates of metabolic syndrome, followed by clozapine, risperidone, and quetiapine. Aripiprazole, lurasidone, and ziprasidone are less likely to cause metabolic syndrome. Therefore, transitioning a patient from clozapine to ziprasidone would be reasonable. Or, a patient could be switched to a typical antipsychotic, which would decrease the metabolic adverse effects but increase the chances of EPS, as discussed previously. Another solution could be to decrease the dose of antipsychotic medication or even stop prescribing the antipsychotic altogether. However, like all other decisions in medicine, the risks and benefits would have to be analyzed. For many patients, antipsychotics facilitate their ability to live safely in the community. Therefore, most patients would rather live with the metabolic complications and increased risk of diabetes and cardiovascular problems than risk hurting themselves or others or have to spend most of their lives in psychiatric institutions.

When a patient develops metabolic syndrome and/or diabetes mellitus (DM), but his or her mental illness is sufficiently burdensome that the antipsychotics cannot be decreased or stopped, the metabolic complications are commonly seen by primary care physicians and can be treated with medications. DM is one of the most common conditions in the United States, and the prevalence is increasing.

There are two types of DM, type I and type II. Type I DM is an autoimmune disorder in which the patient's immune system attacks the cells that produce insulin. These cells, called beta cells, located in the pancreas, are then unable to make insulin, and patients require daily injections of artificial insulin. Type I DM generally starts in childhood. The type of DM that can occur as a result of antipsychotics is type II DM, which results from more long-term damage to pancreatic beta cells. These patients become "insulin resistant," which means that the insulin their bodies produce is unable to function properly. The insulin does not efficiently move glucose from the bloodstream into the cells, so blood sugar gets too high, while cells do not receive proper nourishment. There are many medications available for patients with type II DM.

Most are pills that act in various ways to sensitize the body's cell to insulin, so it can more efficiently do its job. However, when patients' type II DM becomes significantly advanced, they too require daily injections of artificial insulin.

Medications are also widely available to treat high blood pressure and high cholesterol. The most common and effective medications for cholesterol are called statins, which act to prevent the body from synthesizing cholesterol. Statins include brand-name medications like Lipitor (atorvastatin) and Crestor (rosuvastatin). Some physicians recommend prescribing statins to all patients taking antipsychotics as long as there is no contraindication, to prevent them from developing high cholesterol in the first place. However, this practice has not built significant momentum among psychiatrists.

A critical way psychiatrists can address metabolic syndrome in their patients is to work closely and coordinate with other physicians treating the patient. Patient care improves significantly when doctors of various specialties convene to get on the same page regarding a patient's risk factors and what the best options would be from a well-rounded perspective. Psychiatrists should have input from other specialized physicians to understand exactly how problematic a patient's risk factors are and use that contribution to drive the decision-making process.

Antipsychotics and QT Prolongation

As discussed in the previous section, the heart is an organ of particular concern when patients are prescribed antipsychotics. Metabolic syndrome affects the heart's health by leading to damage along blood vessel walls, which can lead to heart attacks or strokes. However, antipsychotics can affect the heart through another mechanism, by disrupting its electrochemical circuits.

Cardiac physiology is complicated and highly specialized. The heart is composed of many muscle fibers that, if working properly, all contract in unison to generate the biggest pump possible. After all, it is the strength of the pump that is going to send blood to every blood vessel in the body, deliver oxygen to all body tissues, and take away all toxic by-products of metabolism. If each muscle fiber in the heart contracted on its own timetable, the heart would not beat hard enough to get this job done. All muscle fibers must contract in synchrony, every beat, 60 to 100 times per minute, on average, 60 minutes per hour, 24 hours per day, 365 days per year, for a nice, long life of 85 years, if we are lucky. To coordinate the teamwork necessary for all 3,574,080,000 beats, the heart relies on a web on electric cables. These bundles comprise the clock that paces the heart. They jump from node to node, and they disseminate to signal each fiber to fire at the exact same time.

Physicians can assess the electric current in the heart with a test called an electrocardiogram (EKG). The test works by placing stickers around the heart that measures the strength of the electric flow in any given direction. The test is painless (except when the technician pulls the stickers off, which is similar to removing a Band-Aid). There are no adverse effects of the test, and it takes about five minutes. The EKG can be divided into sections that correspond with exactly what the heart is doing at any given time, that is, pumping, refilling, and so on. Each segment of the EKG should take a very specific amount of time. Specific points along the cycles of the heartbeat are designated with letters such as P, Q, R, S, T. The length of time between events along the cycle is designated with these letters (e.g., the PR interval or the QT interval). The QT interval roughly represents the period of time during which the ventricles of the heart, the chambers that directly pump blood through the body, contract, pump out the blood, then relax, and refill with blood. This should take between 350 and 450 milliseconds. Antipsychotic medications can lead to an increase in the QT interval, known as QT prolongation, defined as greater than 500 milliseconds.

Many medications cause QT prolongation, including some antibiotics and pain relievers. QT prolongation is generally harmless but can lead to dangerous disruptions in the coordination of heartbeats, known as arrhythmias. The worst outcomes would be an arrhythmia called ventricular fibrillation, which occurs when the muscle fibers in the hearts' ventricles are not operating synchronously. All the fibers are contracting randomly, and the heart is unable to pump blood effectively through the body. This constitutes a medical emergency that is treated with specialized intravenous medications and an electrical shock to the heart to reset and reorganize the electric current. The feared EKG pattern associated with the condition that can lead to ventricular fibrillation is known as "torsades de pointes," which in French roughly means turning around a point. This name comes from the wavy EKG pattern.

The specific link between antipsychotics and sudden cardiac death is controversial. It was first reported in the 1960s and led to greater concern in the 1990s. While one study found that use of antipsychotics, typical and atypical, doubled a patient's risk of sudden cardiac death, it is very difficult, if not impossible, to attribute the condition to the antipsychotics in the setting of many confounding variables. However, physicians agree that increase in the QT interval is a risk factor for adverse cardiac events, and antipsychotics are known to increase the QT interval. The magnitude of that increase depends on a patient's risk factors, the exact antipsychotic used, and the dose of the drug. Higher dosages lead to proportional increases in the QT interval.

There are differences in how psychiatrists understand the risks posed by antipsychotics and QT prolongation. As a result, the way psychiatrists monitor QT prolongation varies among practitioners and settings. Generally, inpatient psychiatrists monitor the QT interval more carefully than outpatient psychiatrists. There are medical and practical reasons behind this trend. Medically, it is more likely for inpatients, patients who are sufficiently psychiatrically unstable to require admission to a hospital, to have more severe psychiatric illnesses, and thus require higher dosages of antipsychotics. Also, many patients admitted to a hospital were not taking antipsychotics prior to admission, so the doses of the antipsychotics are usually increased relatively quickly so that patients can leave the hospital and return to their lives as soon as they are safe. Therefore, the risk of QT prolongation is increased. Practically speaking, it is easier to monitor the QT interval on the inpatient unit than from the outpatient setting, because the patients are there, and they are not going anywhere. A physician can simply call the EKG technician who can perform the EKG the same day. An outpatient physician can refer a patient to a medical office for the test, but the patient is required to take the time to go, which does not happen 100% of the time.

The American Psychiatric Association's practice guidelines do not specifically require routine testing for everyone started on antipsychotics. The guidelines recommend routine EKGs only under several conditions:

- Patients prescribed antipsychotics that have been shown to be more likely to cause QT prolongation, including ziprasidone and thioridazine
- Patients with known abnormalities in the heart rhythm (arrhythmias) or symptoms of arrhythmias, including fainting
- Patients taking other medications that are known to prolong the QT interval, including methadone, an opiate used for pain relief and drug withdrawal, or certain antibiotics such as levofloxacin

However, it is not uncommon for inpatient psychiatrists to establish a baseline EKG prior to initiating antipsychotics and then recheck the EKG each time the dose is significantly increased. There are several circumstances under which concerns about the QT would alter a clinician's practice. Sometimes, particularly in the outpatient setting, patients are not compliant with EKG testing. Due to the nature of schizophrenia, it is possible that arranging an EKG is too difficult for the patient, even with support from the psychiatrist. Alternatively, if patients have cardiac risk factors, or a patient has been shown to have QT prolongation with antipsychotics, the psychiatrist should take that information into account when deciding which medications to choose. Generally, atypical antipsychotics have less QT prolongation, and of the atypicals, aripiprazole and lurasidone are known to affect the QT interval the least.

Constipation

Antipsychotics are notorious for causing constipation. This is largely due to the anticholinergic effects. Therefore, the antipsychotics that have the most anticholinergic activity, including quetiapine, olanzapine, and clozapine, will cause the most constipation.

Constipation is generally considered a minor problem, sometimes causing abdominal discomfort and increased straining during defecation, which could lead to hemorrhoids. However, constipation, if left untreated, can develop into a health crisis. Paralytic ileus is the technical term used when bowels stop moving completely. This can be a fatal condition, often requiring hospitalization and surgery. To avoid this, patients who take antipsychotics should be advised to drink plenty of fluids, eat a high-fiber diet, and exercise regularly. Furthermore, many patients who take antipsychotics are also prescribed laxative medications for daily use. These can range from mild over-the-counter stool softeners to more potent laxatives such as lactulose and polyethylene glycol. Since patients can be embarrassed speaking about this side effect, psychiatrists must directly ask.

Hyperprolactinemia

Prolactin is a hormone that is released from the pituitary gland in the brain into the body. Prolactin has several effects on the body. Although under normal circumstances prolactin's effects are more notable in women, men also synthesize the hormone.

Antipsychotics have an unusual relationship with prolactin. Dopamine typically regulates prolactin in that it has a negative feedback mechanism. The more dopamine in the brain, the less prolactin is released into the body. Dopamine can be thought of as the brakes in the prolactin system. Therefore, when antipsychotics are introduced and block dopamine, the prolactin system is left unchecked. Since it no longer has the brakes, too much prolactin is released into the bloodstream, leading to hyperprolactinemia. Risperidone and paliperidone, for reasons that are not entirely clear, are the antipsychotics most likely to cause hyperprolactinemia. Other antipsychotics implicated in causing hyperprolactinemia are haloperidol and amisulpride.

Men and women experience different effects of hyperprolactinemia. Both genders experience sexual side effects, including decreased libido and an inability to orgasm. Women often have a cessation of menstruation, known as amenorrhea. Men may develop breast tissue, known as gynecomastia, which can be extremely embarrassing. Both genders may even leak fluid from their breasts, called galactorrhea. Infertility can also result from hyperprolactinemia. Symptoms of hyperprolactinemia are generally embarrassing, and patients often do not talk about them with their doctors. Further, routine blood tests to check prolactin levels are not commonly performed. Therefore, patients who are prescribed antipsychotics must be educated about these side effects, and doctors must take the initiative to ask about symptoms so that patients do not have to bring them up if they do not feel comfortable. If patients do report symptoms of hyperprolactinemia, a prolactin blood test is available and can confirm the diagnosis. The recommended treatment strategy would be to switch to an antipsychotic less likely to cause hyperprolactinemia. If a female patient is experiencing amenorrhea and switching antipsychotics is not practical, the medication metformin, typically used to treat DM, has been shown to be effective in restoring menstruation.

Sexual Side Effects

Sexual health is an extremely important component of overall physical and mental health. As discussed earlier, many doctors and patients do not discuss sexual health problems due to embarrassment and discomfort on both sides. Doctors must take the initiative to ask patients about their sexual health. Sexual side effects in patients prescribed antipsychotics are very common. This is due partly to the illness and partly to the treatment. Decreased libido is a symptom in several mental illnesses. However, when appropriately treated, patients with serious mental illnesses often desire and are able to maintain successful, long-term, intimate relationships. In fact, patients in committed relationships have better physical and mental health outcomes than single patients.

Antipsychotics lead to sexual dysfunction through several mechanisms. Antipsychotics decrease dopamine, which, as discussed elsewhere in this text, is the neurotransmitter most associated with pleasure. It is the dopamine rush during sexual activity that makes it a pleasurable experience and encourages people to consistently pursue sexual relationships. When dopamine levels decrease in the brain, the reward feedback is also decreased, leading to a diminished interest in sex. Antipsychotics also block receptors for adrenaline, which is needed for orgasm in both genders. Lastly, antipsychotics lead to hyperprolactinemia, as discussed previously, which exhibits a broad range of effects on sexuality.

According to one study based on patient surveys, 50% of men and 37% of women on antipsychotics reported some degree of sexual dysfunction. Sexual dysfunction can manifest in several ways. Patients can have a decreased libido or desire for sexual relationships. Patients can experience decreased arousal. This can include inability to achieve or maintain erection in men or decreased lubrication or discomfort in women. Patients also suffer from problems with orgasm, either as premature orgasm, delayed orgasm, or inability to achieve orgasm.

There are several strategies to address sexual dysfunction in patients. A psychiatrist can validate and empathetically listen to a patient's concerns. This can result in addressing the shame and embarrassment that often accompany sexual dysfunction. Psychiatrists can also work with the patient and his or her partner to educate them about sexual dysfunction and suggest behavioral solutions. For example, sometimes extended foreplay or the knowledge that sex requires more time accounts for problems with premature or delayed orgasm. Encouraging a partner to adjust his or her sexual routine to create a better experience for a patient may improve libido.

When it is clear that sexual dysfunction can only be addressed with a medication change, psychiatrists can either lower the dose of the medication or switch to a medication that is less likely to cause sexual dysfunction. As mentioned previously, haloperidol, risperidone, paliperidone, and amisulpride are more likely to cause sexual dysfunction, likely because they are more implicated in hyperprolactinemia. Patients can be transitioned to aripirazole, quetiapine, ziprasidone, olanzapine, or clozapine, which are less likely to result in sexual dysfunction.

Neuroleptic Malignant Syndrome

Neuroleptic malignant syndrome (NMS) is a rare but serious adverse effect of antipsychotics. NMS was first described in 1960 and is a condition that involves muscle breakdown. Symptoms include hyperthermia (high fever), rigidity, sweating, blood pressure instability, and altered mental state. Patients suffering from NMS may have fevers as high as 104 or 105 degrees F. Patients can appear confused and progress to coma and, in the most extreme cases, death. NMS is a medical emergency and is treated in intensive care units of the hospitals.

Some antipsychotics are more likely to cause NMS than others. The "high-potency" typical antipsychotics, including haloperidol, are most implicated. However, all antipsychotics have the potential to cause NMS. Studies vary on the exact percentage of patients on antipsychotics that develop NMS. Prevalence rates have been calculated between 0.167 per thousand patients to 32 per thousand patients. While NMS is unpredictable, there are several risk factors that predispose people to the side effect. In terms of the actual medication, patients are more likely to develop NMS when they are first started on antipsychotics, when the dose is increased, when very high dosages are used, or, when more than one antipsychotic is used concurrently. There are conditions patients can be exposed to that make NMS more likely. High temperatures and dehydration put patients more at risk. Further, physical restraint, which should only be used in emergency settings to prevent violence, increases the risk of NMS. Patients who are elderly, have many physical health problems, or have suffered from NMS in the past all have increased rates of NMS.

The exact mechanisms behind NMS are unclear. The dopamine blockade common to all antipsychotics is widely believed to be central in the process. One theory is that dopamine plays a large role in mediating body temperature and muscle tone. Therefore, when dopamine is blocked, the body loses its ability to regulate these systems, and the result is high body temperatures and muscle rigidity. Treatment involves stopping all antipsychotics and administering supportive care, including ice packs, to control the fever and intravenous fluids to stabilize blood pressure. Muscle relaxants, including dantrolene, are also used to help rigidity. Bromocriptine, which acts in the opposite manner as antipsychotics to active dopamine receptors, has been shown to be effective. However, even when recognized, about 10% of NMS cases are fatal. One study found that 11% of atypical-induced NMS and 12% of typical-induced NMS were fatal. As mentioned previously, NMS is very rare, and most psychiatrists have never and will never encounter a patient suffering from the condition.

Clozapine

In several places in this text, the superiority of clozapine has been discussed in its efficacy as a medication. As established by the influential Clinical Antipsychotic Trials of Clinical Effectiveness (CATIE) study in 2005, clozapine therapy improves symptoms of schizophrenia and other psychotic disorders better than other antipsychotics. In fact, clozapine has often been referred to as a "wonder drug" or a "miracle drug." Many psychiatrists have at least one patient for whom clozapine therapy proved invaluable. The typical scenario is that a patient is profoundly disabled and is unable to stay in the community for long stretches of time before being readmitted to a psychiatric hospital. He or she would have taken large doses of many different antipsychotics, sometimes several at a time, without a significant difference.

Then he or she agrees to take clozapine, and his or her family is barely able to recognize their loved one. Clozapine has been shown to be effective for positive and negative symptoms. Therefore, patients are able to stay out of the hospital because the positive symptoms, delusions and hallucinations, no longer make the patient dangerous. And, to the great surprise of the family, patients have improved social skills and are able to work certain jobs due to reduction in negative symptoms. Clozapine is also very inexpensive. It was the first atypical antipsychotic; therefore, the pharmaceutical patent is long expired. Therefore, a reasonable question would be why are not all patients with serious mental illnesses prescribed clozapine? The answer is found in the side effect profile of the drug. Clozapine is arguably the most difficult medication to take in psychiatry and one of the most difficult in all of medicine. It is one of the worst offenders in terms of metabolic syndrome and leads to large weight gain, increase in cholesterol, and increase in the risk of DM. However, probably the most problematic side effect is called clozapine-induced agranulocytosis.

Clozapine-Induced Agranulocytosis

Agranulocytosis is a condition that affects a patient's blood cells. Blood, of course, is a vital part of the body and accomplishes many tasks. It provides all body tissue with oxygen and nutrition and carries away all by-products and waste of metabolism. Other parts of the blood, called white blood cells, lead the body's immune response. They fight unwelcome intruders, including viruses, bacteria, fungi, cancer, and the like. The mechanisms these cells use to recognize intruders, kill them, and remember them for the next time they come around are one of the complicated aspects of biochemistry. Within white bloods cells (WBCs), there are many type of cells that specialize in targeting different types of attackers. A WBC line called lymphocytes primarily target viruses, and granulocytes, also called neutrophils, target bacteria. Clozapine has the side effect of decreasing the number of granulocytes in the blood, hence the name, agranulocytosis. This leaves the body susceptible to potentially lethal bacterial infections. As mentioned elsewhere, the discovery that clozapine can cause this side effect, first reported in the 1970s in Finland, almost led to clozapine's disappearance from the market. However, physicians appreciated that clozapine was incredibly valuable to many patients, and clozapine-induced agranulocytosis can be detected before it poses a significant danger. Therefore, clozapine remained part of psychiatrists' arsenal to fight serious mental illnesses, but strict guidelines were introduced to avoid serious illness and death due to clozapine-induced agranulocytosis.

The basic way to safely administer clozapine is to monitor patients' blood through frequent laboratory tests called complete blood count (CBC). CBCs are very common lab tests. Essentially all doctors look at all patients' CBCs during both routine check-ups and when patients are ill. CBCs reveal infections, anemia, certain cancers, and a host of other medical problems. CBCs are broken down to allow the doctor to see the exact level of each type of cell in the blood. This way, doctors can notice when granulocytes, or neutrophils, are decreasing, and they can stop clozapine long before patients are at risk.

There is a very specific blood-monitoring regimen that is required for patients taking clozapine. Patients get weekly CBCs for six months, then CBCs every two weeks for six months, then monthly CBCs indefinitely. Therefore, even if a patient has taken clozapine for 30 years without any WBC abnormality, he or she still must get a CBC every month. Further, if there is a disruption in the clozapine therapy and the patient stops taking it for even several days, the blood monitoring must restart from the beginning, because the chances of agranulocytosis would be equal to that of a patient starting initially. There are times when even the most diligent and responsible clozapine patients are unable to access their medications. For example, they may be on vacation and a suitcase is lost by an airline. Or, they may have a serious medical problem and doctors at a hospital may not know to give the patient clozapine. This is very frustrating to patients because they then have to have weekly and biweekly CBCs for an entire year.

There are specific guidelines that psychiatrists follow depending on the results of the laboratory blood tests:

- Healthy patients have WBCs greater than 3,500 per cubic millimeter or absolute neutrophil count (ANC) greater than 2,000 per cubic millimeter. The ANC is more important than the general WBC. Patients with these values can continue taking clozapine normally.
- Patients with ANC values of 1,500–2,000 have mild granulocytopenia, and monitoring should be increased to twice weekly.
- Patients with ANC values of 1,000–1,500 have moderate granulocytopenia, and clozapine therapy should be suspended until neutrophil count returns to normal. Once clozapine is started, monitoring should be weekly, as with any patient starting the medication.
- Patients with ANC values of below 1,000 have agranulocytosis. These patients are at high risk of serious infection, and clozapine therapy should be stopped and never started again.

Agranulocytosis occurs in approximately 0.8% of cases (8 in 1,000). The risk for WBC dysfunction is highest early in treatment, about 6 to 18 months after clozapine is started. Rates of mortality in patients who have documented clozapine-induced agranulocytosis range from 2% to 20%. Lithium, a commonly used mood stabilizer, has the opposite effect on WBCs as clozapine. Lithium causes a proliferation of WBCs, with patients frequently showing higher levels. If necessary, psychiatrists can prescribe lithium to increase a patient's WBCs to make them eligible for clozapine therapy.

This blood monitoring is a necessary but enormous barrier to treatment with clozapine. Weekly blood draws are time-consuming, inconvenient, and painful. This component of taking a medication would be a difficult sell to even someone without any mental illness, but considering that clozapine is used in the most extreme cases of psychosis, it is easy to understand why this therapy is underutilized. Patients do not want to make that commitment and often do not attend appointments at the laboratory.

This blood monitoring is carefully recorded in a clozapine registry at clozapinerems.com. The registry compiles all laboratory results from all patients who are given clozapine. This is important because patients with serious mental illnesses often are not able to provide detailed histories of their treatment. If a patient experiences agranulocytosis with clozapine and then goes to another provider, even in another state, that provider will see the patient's history with clozapine and will be unable to prescribe the drug. The clozapine registry is also linked to pharmacies that distribute clozapine. The doctor is required to enter the results of the patient's CBC, which the pharmacy needs to dispense the medication. Without the appropriate laboratory work, pharmacies are not permitted to distribute clozapine. For example, if a new clozapine patient has a normal CBC, the psychiatrist can only prescribe one week of clozapine. If the doctor makes a mistake and gives the patient a prescription for one month, the pharmacy will not fill that prescription.

This level of scrutiny is unique to clozapine-induced agranulocytosis. For example, patients who take any antipsychotic should get laboratory tests for DM and cholesterol every three months. However, if patients do not go to the lab to get these tests, which is frequent, psychiatrists can use their discretion and continue to prescribe antipsychotics if they think the benefits outweigh the risks of continuing treatment. However, psychiatrists cannot use their discretion with clozapine. If the CBC is not received by a pharmacy through the clozapine registry, the psychiatrist is unable to use clozapine.

Clozapine-Induced Myocarditis

Another serious and potentially fatal side effect of clozapine is myocarditis. Myocarditis is essentially an inflammation of the muscle fibers that make up the heart. Myocarditis is rare, occurring in 0.2–1% of patients prescribed clozapine. Symptoms generally appear within the first months of treatment and initially include a flu-like illness, with generally malaise, fatigue, diarrhea, and painful urination. Later, patients experience chest pain, tachycardia, fever, and signs of heart failure.

It is impossible to predict which patients will develop clozapine-induced myocarditis. Unlike with clozapine-induced agranulocytosis, there is no laboratory test that can reliably detect its presence before the patient is in danger. Patients must be educated about clozapine-induced myocarditis so that if they do develop symptoms, they know to go to an emergency room immediately and explain to doctors what may be happening. Blood tests that look for heart muscle breakdown in the blood, in addition to specific EKG findings, can confirm the diagnosis. The treatment is to immediately stop clozapine. Anti-inflammatory agents, including nonsteroidal anti-inflammatory drugs (NSAIDs) like ibuprofen and steroids, such as prednisone, are frequently used. Once a patient has experienced clozapine-induced myocarditis, he or she should never be given another trial of clozapine again.

Clozapine-Induced Seizures

There is a correlation between seizures and high-dose clozapine use. This effect is typically seen at doses over 600 mg daily. Typical doses are 200–800 mg total daily. The chances of seizures are 1% for doses lower than 300 mg daily, 2.7% for doses between 300 and 600 mg daily, and 4.4% for dosages greater than 600 mg. When seizures do occur, the recommended approach is to lower the dose. When this is accomplished, seizures generally stop. If it is not safe to lower the dose of clozapine for psychiatric reasons, patients can be given antiepileptic medication, normally prescribed to patients with seizure disorders.

Excessive Salivation

Excessive salivation, or sialorrhea, can be a side effect of any antipsychotic, but it is mostly seen with clozapine. Patients typically experience symptoms at night, often waking up with a wet pillow. This symptom can be embarrassing and also leads to disrupted sleep. The mechanism of this side effect is thought to be both increased saliva production and decreased swallowing. Because this side effect does not have significant health consequences, it is typically not a reason psychiatrists will change from clozapine to another antipsychotic. However, if patients are sufficiently bothered by the drooling and it poses an obstacle to medication compliance, psychiatrists must take it seriously. There are several medications that can counter this side effect, including glycopyrrolate, benztropine, and clonidine.

Disclosing Side Effects of Antipsychotics

One very challenging question faced by all physicians is how to talk to patients about medication side effects. Every medication, including over-the-counter pain medications like acetaminophen and ibuprofen, has long lists of possible side effects. Therefore, how would a doctor know which side effects to discuss with patients? Psychiatrists have an even more complex challenge, given the nature of their patients' illnesses. Many psychiatric patients are already skeptical of medications, especially patients with psychotic illnesses who are generally paranoid. Psychiatrists fear that by disclosing the long lists of side effects, patients will refuse the medications they need.

The topic of exactly what doctors should disclose has been the subject of several legal cases, after patients who developed side effects sued doctors because they did not believe they were told the whole story about specific medications. In 1955, a woman name Irma Natanson was diagnosed with breast cancer and received treatment at a hospital in Kansas. During the treatment, she suffered from radiation burns that were a known side effect of the treatment but were never disclosed to her by the physician, Dr. John Kline. In the case that followed, *Natanson v. Kline* (1960), the Kansas Supreme Court decided that physicians have an obligation to disclose only what the typical reasonable doctor would say to his or her patients. Twelve years after that ruling, a court in Washington, DC, changed the established practice in the case *Canterbury v. Spence* (1972). Mr. Canterbury fell after a back surgery performed by Dr. Spence due to swelling of the spinal cord and was not told of such a risk. The court changed the standard, making it a requirement that doctors disclose what the typical reasonable patient would want to know, instead of just what the typical doctor would want to explain.

Therefore, as a result of courts' decisions, across all fields of medicine, doctors are expected to tell patients everything the "reasonable" patient would want to know before starting a medication. How do doctors translate that into actual practice? It is unreasonable to expect doctors to go through every side effect of every medication in detail. If that were the accepted practice, the entire doctor's appointment would be spent discussing side effects that will most likely never occur. Further, patients would not want to take the medications that they need to treat serious medical conditions. Therefore, many doctors highlight the most commonly occurring side effects. It is not expected for doctors to detail side effects that occur only in extremely rare circumstances, unless that side effect is very severe. For example, NMS is extremely rare, but it can cause death. Therefore, despite its infrequency, the "reasonable person" would want to know about a potentially lethal side effect, so it should be disclosed. Different psychiatrists practice differently. However, most would agree that when patients begin taking antipsychotics, psychiatrists would be expected to tell them about increased risk of weight gain, DM, increased blood pressure, increased cholesterol, movement disorders, and NMS.

Because antipsychotics have significant adverse effects, psychiatrists must carefully consider whether the risks of giving the medications outweigh the benefits. If they believe the medications are appropriate, psychiatrists must carefully explain the side effects and also teach the patient about the illness and the risks of *not* taking medications, including paranoid delusions, hallucinations, and significant social and occupational impairment. After the psychiatrist has explained why the benefits of treatment outweigh the risks, he or she must teach the patient how the side effects will be monitored and addressed. It is important for the patient to know that the psychiatrist will order laboratory tests on a frequent basis that show trends in glucose metabolism and cholesterol. This way, if metabolic side effects do occur, the patient and the psychiatrist can address the situation before the patient suffers any major health problems. Of course, when patients hear that the medication can cause death as a result of NMS, many patients resist treatment. They should be made aware that this is an extremely rare occurrence, and, if given proper and timely medical care, the condition is treatable.

However, it is possible, and happens often, that after a full disclosure of the side effects, patients who truly need antipsychotics decide they do not want to take them, as is their right. As discussed elsewhere in this text, there are very specific times when patients can be compelled to take antipsychotics, but in the vast majority of cases, even profoundly ill patients have the right to decide not to take antipsychotics, both in the community and in the hospital. It is important for physicians to be comfortable with the idea that patients have autonomy over their bodies, and they have the right to make choices that are medically unwise. Doctors should be able to continue working with patients in a professional manner despite the disagreement and collaborate with them about other therapies to which they would consent.

MISUSE OF ANTIPSYCHOTICS

The risks associated with the misuse of antipsychotics are much different than those of other classes of medications. Medications or drugs have the potential for widespread abuse when they have effects that are outside the indications of their prescription. Many common drugs of abuse were originally developed by pharmaceutical companies, or their precursors, to address a medical problem. Opium-based painkillers, like Percocet or Vicodin, are synthesized from the same base substance as heroin. While these medications accomplish their intended purpose of significantly relieving pain, their widespread abuse has become a major public health concern because they also can cause a euphoric state and are highly addictive. Other medications, like synthetic hormones, have the secondary effect of facilitating rapid muscle growth, leading to abuse in athletes and many image-conscious men.

Antipsychotics are generally unlike these medications, in that abusing them serves little purpose. Put another way, taking antipsychotics is not *fun*. Instead of making people feel happy and disinhibited like most substances of abuse, antipsychotics cause people to feel fatigued, sleepy, and physically stiff. Instead of allowing users to have a potentially attractive physique, like anabolic steroids, antipsychotics cause weight gain. And instead of leading to enhanced sexual performance, like the frequently recreationally used Viagra and similar medications, antipsychotics cause impotence and decreased libido. Therefore, people rarely take antipsychotics unless prescribed by a physician to treat a serious mental illness. The one exception is the antipsychotic quetiapine (Seroquel). As discussed elsewhere in this text, quetiapine has high anticholinergic properties, which cause some light-headedness, that some people find rewarding. Currently, many jails and prisons do not prescribe inmates quetiapine because of the potential black-market resale value and abuse potential. Other than that, there is no noteworthy secondary market in antipsychotics. Drug dealers on the corner may hawk painkillers and antianxiety medications in addition to the normal substances of abuse, but they probably would not sell antipsychotics because there is not much demand.

ANTIPSYCHOTIC OVERDOSE AND TOXICITY

Antipsychotic overdoses are unfortunately common because the patients who take antipsychotics suffer from illnesses that are associated with suicide. Antipsychotics are most often prescribed to patients with schizophrenia, schizoaffective disorder, and bipolar disorder, which carry completed suicide rates of between 10% and 20%. The attempted suicide rates for these illnesses are much higher, and one of the most common methods is medication overdose. Therefore, all properly trained psychiatrists and emergency room physicians are aware of the symptoms of antipsychotic toxicity.

Antipsychotic overdoses are rarely fatal. This is due to the fact that the effects of overdose are generally uncomfortable but not extremely dangerous.

While many overdoses are the method of many attempted suicides, completed suicides are much more likely to occur with self-inflicted gunshot wounds or asphyxiation. The precise symptoms of antipsychotic toxicity vary among different medications. However, in general, symptoms of overdose are caused by the anticholinergic (blocks acetylcholine), antihistaminergic (blocks histamine), and antiadrenergic (block adrenaline) properties of antipsychotics.

Excessive anticholinergic substances will cause confusion, blurry vision, constipation, difficulty urinating, and dry mouth, in addition to other symptoms. Toxic levels of antihistaminergic drugs will cause somnolence and fatigue. Overdoses of antiadrenergic compounds will cause a slowed heart rate (bradycardia) and dizziness when standing up due to a sharp decrease in blood pressure (orthostatic hypotension). Therefore, someone who just ingested an entire bottle of antipsychotic in a suicide attempt may be dizzy and confused. They may not be able to focus on the doctor because they cannot see well. When they try to stand up, they may fall due to orthostatic hypotension. They may have difficulty annunciating due to a dry mouth (and confusion).

The most dangerous results of an antipsychotic overdose are the cardiac implications. Antipsychotics cause a slowing, or disruption, of the electrical circuits of the heart. The heartbeats are based on electrical signals that originate in centers (nodes) and then travel throughout the cardiac tissue. This occurs rhythmically and highly consistently. Antipsychotics can cause the signal to slow down and in extreme cases, to be interrupted. If this occurs, the individual muscle fibers of the heart cease to pump in unison, and blood will not be efficiently ejected from the heart's chambers into the body. This can lead to death, but it is a very rare occurrence in antipsychotic toxicity.

Therefore, the best way to treat overdosed patients is to treat their symptoms and monitor them. Of course, physicians will also stop administering antipsychotic drugs until they are without symptoms of toxicity. Intravenous hydration will address the orthostatic hypotension, dry mouth, and blurriness. After several hours, or over several days, the symptoms can be expected to subside. Overdosed patients are usually monitored with a continuous EKG called telemetry for at least 24 hours to detect any of the dangerous cardiac changes.

Chapter 7

Production, Distribution, and Regulation

This chapter will cover some of the logistics behind making the medications and distributing them throughout the country and the world. For those interested in the more clinical aspects of the medications, there might be some question as to the importance of this information. In the following pages, the information provided will be not only giving information about how the production and distribution are managed but also what clinical and ethical implications should be understood when gaining insight into the business behind the creation of any product, especially when it is a product that will be consumed by the targeted population. This chapter will start with an overview of the pharmaceutical industry in general and then look a little closer at pharmaceutical companies responsible for some of the already mentioned antipsychotics. It will explore the Food and Drug Administration's (FDA) process of approval as well as specific antipsychotics that have been approved but have other regulatory agencies involved in their distribution and finally will look at some regulations that are not federally mandated, but that many clinics utilize.

PHARMACEUTICAL INDUSTRY

The short story is that pharmaceutical companies develop, test, produce, and market drugs to be used as medications. They are subject to a number of different regulatory organizations and processes as they travel through the development and production of a drug. The medication that they market can be sold as either a brand-name medication or a generic medication. A brand-name medication is a drug that has been approved for a patent. The pharmaceutical company that developed and produced the drug applies for a patent in order to protect against other companies making copies of the medication and selling the drug. A generic drug is a copy of one of those branded medications. The generic medication contains the active ingredient that has already been approved by the FDA and they are not patented. Generally, the pharmaceutical company that is developing the new drug has funded the research and development of the new branded drug on its own and this is not cheap. So, when they market a new branded medication, the cost of the medication is high in order to cover the costs they underwent in order to create it and still make a profit. The generic medication is usually much cheaper than the branded medication because it is using an active ingredient that has already been approved by the FDA, so the cost for development and production is much lower than that for a newly patented medication. Thus far, all of this information seems to be just about how these companies operate in relation to each other, trying to develop new medications and also trying to make money; but how does this affect the consumer of the medication, the patient? The issue for the consumer comes into play when looking at availability of the generic medication. This is the cheaper of the medications, making it the most accessible to the majority of the population. However, the generic medication, using the same active ingredient as the branded medication, cannot become available to the public until the branded medication's patent expires. The length of the patent is different from drug to drug based on a number of variables but is generally years and can be up to 20 years, meaning that people are often forced to pay higher prices or use a less desirable medication while waiting for the patent to expire and a generic form to become available. Later in the chapter there will be examples of antipsychotics and the difference in cost between branded and generic medications, but on average the generic medication is 80–85% cheaper than the branded medication. It is no secret these days that the pharmaceutical industry is a big business that is interested in making money and has been very successful in doing that, and antipsychotic development is no exception.

The history of the pharmaceutical industry is long and complicated. It has roots that trace back all the way to the 1660s, with Merck, now ranked the third largest pharmaceutical company in the world by *Forbes* in 2015 with $11.9 billion in profits in 2015, that began as a small apothecary shop in 1668 in Germany. The other half to the history is roots that trace back to chemical companies that had research labs and discovered medical applications for products in the 1880s. Eventually these two paths crossed and merged to combine the development of the product, production, application, and distribution. It is important to have some understanding of the history of organizations creating a product because it helps to understand some of their motives in marketing. Over the past few decades there have been big changes in how pharmaceutical companies are received in the clinical setting, which will be discussed further later in the chapter, as it has ethical and clinical practice implications. However, first it is important to have some understanding of the regulatory body governing the development and production of all medications.

Food and Drug Administration

Commonly referred to as the FDA, the Food and Drug Administration is a federal agency of the U.S. Department of Health and Human Services. Its mission is to promote public health through regulation and supervision of a variety of products, often those that are consumed by the population or their pets. The organization has an extremely wide range of areas of oversee, including, but not limited to, supplements, tobacco, food, veterinary products, and prescription and over-the-counter pharmaceutical drugs, most applicable to this book.

The FDA regulates nearly every aspect of prescription drugs, including testing, manufacturing, labeling, advertising, marketing, safety, and efficacy, which means that the pharmaceutical companies and their processes are very closely linked and intertwined with the FDA and its regulatory processes. The regulatory agency is designed to make sure that the drug being developed is safe, efficacious, and marketed properly to the general public and providers. As mentioned previously, medications that are used "on-label" are medications that have been FDA-approved to treat a specific symptom or disease. Generally speaking, this means that the medication has been researched, developed, and tested to treat a specific disease and has been found safe enough and effective enough to be marketed to treat that disease. On the other hand, sometimes doctors prescribe medications "off-label," which means that they have not been FDA-approved for that specific symptom or disease. So what does it take to get a medication FDA-approved? This is where our pharmaceutical companies overlap with the regulatory agencies in order to attempt to create a product that is beneficial, safe, and profitable.

The FDA has a branch, Center for Drug Evaluation and Research, which is solely devoted to the regulation of drug production. The mission of this branch is to ensure that drugs that are marketed in the United States are safe and effective. The steps can be viewed generally rather simply and divided into two main steps. First, the pharmaceutical company does all of the research, development, and proposal for product labeling. They need to ensure that they have done enough research to support that the proposed medication will be relatively safe and effective in treating humans. The word "relatively" is important, because as mentioned previously, when considering use of medications, one must always think about it as a risk versus benefit ratio, as no medication is without side effects and few are fully efficacious. This development process takes years of work done by many people and a large monetary sum to fund the project. Once it is prepared, the pharmaceutical company submits a new drug application to the FDA to be reviewed in an attempt to get their approval. The second step is the FDA review. A team of physicians, statisticians, chemists, pharmacologists, and other scientists working for the Center for Drug Evaluation and Research will review the submission and consider the data to support the use of the medication as well as how they have labeled and marketed the drug. It will then be either approved or not approved. If the drug is not approved, the FDA will explain why and will inform the company of what would need to be done differently or further research necessary in order to get approval. This explanation is a simplified version of the process, which takes years, often some back and forth between the company and regulatory agency, and millions of dollars. All of the antipsychotics that have been mentioned have gone through this process and received some type of FDA approval. Some of the individual medications and their approval and regulation will be discussed in detail in the following pages.

Johnson and Johnson

According to *Forbes*, which considers revenues, profits, assets, and market value, Johnson and Johnson was the world's largest drug company for the year 2015. Janssen Pharmaceuticals is a subsidiary company of Johnson and Johnson that is responsible for the production and approval of Risperdal, Risperdal Consta, and Invega. As mentioned previously, the description above is a simplified one and the path to getting approval and then finding other drugs to market as well is more complicated. The next paragraphs will explore that journey with Janssen, Johnson and Johnson, Risperdal, and Invega.

Risperdal is the brand name for the active ingredient and generic medication, risperidone. It was the second atypical antipsychotic to be introduced to the U.S. market, after clozapine, and was FDA-approved in 1993 to treat schizophrenia in adults. As mentioned earlier in the book, Risperdal is now approved to treat many other disorders and age groups, including, but not limited to, bipolar disorder, irritability in autism, and schizophrenia for the pediatric population. The approvals for all of these other disorders came at different times throughout the life of Risperdal, most recently getting FDA approval in 2007. Janssen Pharmaceuticals also developed a long-acting injectable form of Risperdal called Risperdal Consta that was FDA-approved for the treatment of schizophrenia in 2003. The original new drug application was submitted in

August 2001, and the FDA responded with an action letter in June 2002 with actions that needed to be taken prior to approval. Then between April and the end of October 2003, Janssen submitted amendments to the original application eight times before it was reviewed and finally approved at the end of October 2003. This highlights some of the obstacles that companies may face when trying to get approval for a medication. All of this work costs a lot of time and money for a company. Sometimes this leads to companies not attempting to get FDA approval for a certain use, especially if it already has approval for a different use, because the cost is just too high, even though based on mechanism of action and clinical experience, it would likely be approved. This leads to more medications being used "off-label" because it would just be too expensive and not profitable to actually get FDA approval.

This also is starting to show a trend that is popular among pharmaceutical companies in order to continue to make a large profit. Risperdal was first approved in 1993, and 10 years later they got approval for the same active ingredient, only in a long-acting injectable form, which would be a patented medication. Risperdal's patent was set to expire in December 2007, and in December 2006, Janssen had Invega FDA-approved. Invega is an extended-release formulation of paliperidone, which is the major active metabolite of Risperdal, meaning that when Risperdal is metabolized in the body, it creates an active product called paliperidone. This active metabolite was developed into the drug Invega, which targets the same disorders that Risperdal does. Many suggested that this was a "patent extender," meaning that Janssen developed this new medication knowing that one of their big moneymakers, Risperdal, was going to become available in a generic form soon. So, in order to continue to be able to make large profits without developing an entirely new medication, a very similar medication is developed that then will extend time under patent for basically the same active ingredient. Not surprisingly, Janssen Pharmaceuticals was also the company responsible for development and marketing of Haldol, one of the most used typical antipsychotics, and in the 1980s, Johnson and Johnson's biggest moneymaking drug. To be clear, Johnson and Johnson is not the only pharmaceutical company that is regularly working to develop new drugs or use similar active ingredients in order to increase profits. Next we will take a look at another pharmaceutical, Otsuka, operating in a similar fashion with the active ingredient aripiprazole.

Otsuka

Otsuka is an international pharmaceutical company based in Japan that is responsible for the development and production of the atypical antipsychotic Abilify. Recall from before that this medication is unique as it was the first to both block dopamine in some areas and increase dopamine in other areas. Abilify was originally approved by the FDA in 2002 and has been an extremely profitable medication for Otsuka. From 2011 to 2012 Abilify generated some $5.4 billion in revenue for the company. The antipsychotic market in pharmaceuticals remains a huge driver of business and not for just one or two companies. It has become clear that there are incredibly large profits accessible in this industry, and pharmaceutical companies are trying to get their foot in the door however they can. Abilify also has a disintegrating tablet form that has been approved for use by the FDA. However, this was not produced solely by Otsuka. This form of the medication was developed, produced, and marketed by Bristol-Myers Squibb in conjunction with Otsuka, which is the same pharmaceutical company that produced and marketed Prolixin. In October 2014, the patent on Abilify expired, and in April 2015, the first generic version, aripiprazole, was FDA-approved, making aripiprazole more widely accessible. This is projected to hurt profits for both Otsuka and Bristol-Myers—the latter also markets for Abilify in conjunction with Otsuka, tremendously.

As Otsuka is losing one of their biggest moneymakers, if they follow the same pattern that was seen with Johnson and Johnson, then they should be looking to develop a similar drug that they can then patent and market much better or with fewer side effects than Abilify. In July 2015, the FDA announced the approval of Rexulti for the treatment of schizophrenia in adults. The active ingredient in Rexulti is brexpiprazole, and the drug was developed and is marketed by Otsuka. The medication is considered to be the successor of Abilify and has a similar mechanism of action. It is presumed that Abilify (aripiprazole) works by blocking some serotonin and dopamine receptors and increasing serotonin and dopamine at other receptors. Rexulti (brexpiprazole) is presumed to work by blocking some serotonin receptors and increasing serotonin and dopamine at other receptors. This is just one of many examples of a pharmaceutical company taking one active ingredient and developing a medication utilizing a very similar active ingredient and getting a new patent.

This is the way of the pharmaceutical industry and by no means is this limited to just psychotropic medications; the same pattern of business stretches across antibiotics, antihypertensives, and medications to lower cholesterol, to name a few. To recap what has been discussed in the previous pages, the pharmaceutical industry is a multibillion dollar industry that is consistently working to develop and market new medications. They are regulated by the FDA and have to get approval in order to market for a specific treatment. There are many steps to go through in order to get a medication on the market, and the goal of the pharmaceuticals is profit. Some of the ways that they attempt to maintain profit were illustrated above using Johnson and Johnson and Otsuka as examples. There is no way around the pharmaceutical companies and their role in drug development, which leads to the question of how much their marketing can be trusted.

There is no clear, black and white answer to this; however, there have been plenty of lawsuits regarding marketing of medications to suggest that at the very least, one should have a healthy skepticism and be curious about the motives of the company in their drug development. Two examples of this in the antipsychotic industry will be covered next, but again, this is not a problem with pharmaceutical companies and antipsychotics but stretches across all different classes of medications.

In 2013, Johnson and Johnson settled in court with the government and agreed to pay $2.2 billion in criminal and civil fines to settle accusations that it improperly promoted Risperdal. Johnson and Johnson pled guilty to a criminal misdemeanor, acknowledging that it improperly marketed Risperdal to the elderly for unapproved uses. More specifically, it was being marketed toward elderly patients with dementia, especially in nursing home settings, even though they had evidence that there could be increased risk of things like stroke in the elderly with dementia. The civil portion of the settlement addresses the company's promotion of Risperdal for people with mental disabilities and children prior to 2006 when they received FDA approval for those populations. The federal government stated that the company knew the risks of weight gain, increased blood sugar level, and increased prolactin level, but they marketed them to providers who served children as safe, without acknowledging those risks.

In 2010, AstraZeneca (manufacturer of Seroquel) denied allegations made but still settled in a civil suit brought about by federal and state entities, agreeing to pay $520 million. The investigation was brought about by a whistle-blower lawsuit with allegations that the company promoted Seroquel to providers between 2001 and 2006 for disorders not covered by FDA approval. The suit also included allegations about kickbacks, which in the pharmaceutical world are payments made to providers or organizations to use or promote their medication. AstraZeneca was accused of "improperly and unduly" influencing company-sponsored continuing medical education programs, which was considered a violation of the Anti-Kickback Statute. This is a federal statute designed to protect patients and federal health-care programs from fraud and abuse by limiting the financial incentives that could be provided by manufacturing firms to induce or reward a certain type of health care.

Both of these examples highlight some of the most complicated aspects of the production and regulation of all medications, including antipsychotics.

The regulatory agencies are in place and designed to approve medications only for uses that have been shown to be beneficial with a relatively acceptable amount of risk. The FDA is even designed to monitor and regulate how a drug can be marketed and who it can be marketed to. Yet the pharmaceutical industry, sometimes referred to as Big Pharma, is a large, wealthy, and influential entity, which by its nature is difficult to regulate. The above examples show how Big Pharma attempts to work around some of those regulations in order to make their drug more profitable. They also show that the government is attempting still to regulate that, but at times it does not happen in the moment and instead occurs after the fact with a lawsuit. So where is Big Pharma today and what is its relationship like with psychiatry?

Pharmaceuticals and Psychiatry

The psychiatric industry has been criticized in the past as one of the leading medical industries in accepting Pharma funding. However, the criticism in accepting funding or gifts from the pharmaceuticals has been slowly developing over the past few decades. Pharmaceutical companies have had drug reps coming to doctors' offices, medical schools, academic hospitals, and the like for years and years and it was accepted readily. In the past few decades, this has been questioned and become frowned upon. This idea stems from the federal statute against kickbacks. The thought is that if the pharmaceutical companies are paying for lunches, buying gifts, or sending prescribers on trips, they may be more likely to prescribe the medication they are promoting. For years physicians have responded to this by suggesting that just because they are receiving monetary benefits from an organization that does not mean it impacts what medications they prescribe. Some physicians will even still argue this. However, the evidence says otherwise. Multiple studies have shown that physicians who receive "perks" from a drug representative show a change in their prescribing patterns to prescribe that medication more often than physicians who do not receive those same perks. Since studies like this have become more prevalent, the attitude toward Big Pharma funding or gifting, even for smaller examples like a free lunch, pen, or sample, has shifted. However, there is still some criticism toward the psychiatric field suggesting that the pharmaceutical companies have too much sway, effecting overall clinical practice in general.

One of the reasons that the relationship between Big Pharma and psychiatry has been so entwined over the past few decades is because of the increase in psychotropic use over that time period. The American Psychiatric Association (APA) suggests that part of that perception is because psychiatry and Big

Pharma have been working together to help sensitize the public to the reality of mental illness. However, they acknowledge that the two entities, Big Pharma and the psychiatric industry, have two very different motives which can be conflictual. For that reason, there is continued push to keep or remove Big Pharma from forums that allow them to influence a physician's prescribing practice.

All of the previously mentioned information about pharmaceutical companies, the FDA and the various problems with regulation and promotion give a basic understanding for how a medication is developed and marketed. This is important to a person as a patient and potential consumer because it is useful to be informed and feel comfortable asking questions to your doctor if you do not understand a medication choice. Information about the production, regulation, and marketing helps to empower patients to help make good health-care decisions for themselves in collaboration with a physician.

The regulation discussed above only applies to the United States. However, the FDA does have a globalization initiative to address the challenge of making sure that imported drugs are regulated and will be safe and effective. It attempts to do this by having arrangements with foreign counterpart regulatory authorities to share information as well as having staff in certain overseas regions. Other countries have their own counterpart national regulatory agencies to ensure that medications that are marketed and sold in their nation are safe and effective but are too extensive to be covered in this book. Thus far, this has been an examination of the regulation of the production of medications in this country in general with some focus on the field of psychiatry. The next pages will take a look at some of the more specific regulations on antipsychotics.

ANTIPSYCHOTICS IN NURSING HOMES

In 2012, the Centers for Medicare and Medicaid Services (CMS) Office of Clinical Standards and Quality issued a nursing home action plan. The aim of the action plan was to improve U.S. health care focusing on three objectives: improving the individual experience of care, improving the health of populations, and reducing the per capita cost of care. The plan uses five actionable strategies, one of which is to promote quality improvement. Under this strategy there was an initiative to address what was called an inappropriate use of antipsychotic medications in nursing homes. The CMS noted that antipsychotics are frequently prescribed off-label to residents with dementia in order to manage behavioral and psychological symptoms. They noted that nursing home residents are often medically complex and at risk for adverse events due to polypharmacy. They suggest that the use of the antipsychotics points to a larger problem, being that nursing homes do not have a systematic plan to provide comprehensive behavioral health management, and so often they turn to antipsychotics. In accordance with the plan, the CMS initially did studies to examine and report on the use of antipsychotics in nursing homes across the country in order to develop quality measures and indicators to enhance the performance metric. The CMS set an initial goal of an average of a 15% reduction in antipsychotic use in nursing homes across the country. Their initial target was to ensure that rapid progress was made and a solid infrastructure was put in place. The goal was that a system should be put in place, and each facility should work with a pharmacy vendor and consultant pharmacist to identify residents on antipsychotics. Then each person should be examined by an interdisciplinary treating team to determine whether that dose could be reduced or discontinued. The CMS has attempted to regulate and decrease the use of antipsychotics in nursing homes in a variety of ways; however, most of them have to do with reporting use and have been largely unsuccessful thus far.

The attempts to regulate use in nursing homes were initially targeted at simply pointing out the problem and beginning an initiative to decrease it. The goal for reduction was not met in 2013. Between 2014 and 2015 antipsychotic use in long-term and short-term residents was added to one of the CMS quality measure domains that impact the scoring system for nursing homes. By including this information in a quality measure the CMS gets reports on the percentage of residents being prescribed antipsychotics during a target period. This information is then added into a formula that is used in a point system to determine a star rating for nursing homes. The idea behind this seems to be that nursing homes would have pressure to reduce antipsychotic use in order to attempt to increase their star rating. The star rating has been used by Medicare for the past five years and not only does have some impact on bonus payments and rebates for enrollees but also works to attract potential families and residents to nursing homes with higher ratings and likely deters people from using nursing homes with lower star ratings. Thus far, this attempt to regulate antipsychotics in nursing homes has also been largely unsuccessful; however, the CMS continues to try to improve their monitoring, quality measures, and performance improvement in order to regulate their use.

PRIOR AUTHORIZATION

The above is an example of an attempt to regulate antipsychotic use due to concern for their safety and risk of adverse effects on patients; prior authorization is another form of regulation with a twofold purpose. Prior authorization is a process used by many health insurance companies, including Medicare and

Medicaid, to determine if they will cover costs of a certain health-care procedure or medication. It is intended to assist in cost-saving for health care in general as well as provide a safety check. However, it is not standardized across the country or by insurance companies and has been criticized for many aspects of the process. Often times the process is required to be manual, can take hours of work by the physician, and sometimes takes up to 30 days for approval, which can lead to a lapse in treatment. It has been estimated that current prior authorization practices cost the U.S. health-care system somewhere between $20 and $30 billion per year.

Prior authorization applies to all types of medications, including antipsychotics, yet as mentioned previously there is no standardization. Each insurance company has its own list of preferred medications and medications that require prior authorization. Generally, medications that are newer, still on patent, and more expensive require prior authorization. When requesting prior authorization, insurance companies are generally interested in making sure the medication requested is being used for an FDA-approved diagnosis. They also gather information about what other medications have been tried and why they were unsuccessful. Prior authorization has the potential to be a way to monitor medication use for safety purposes. It seems that most often, the goal of prior authorization is to reduce costs of insurance company spending on medication. However, this could be an area of development in the future to guide antipsychotic and other medication use in an efficacious and safe way. There is currently strict regulation to monitor one of the antipsychotics to ensure patient safety, which will be discussed in the next pages.

THE UNIQUE CASE OF CLOZAPINE

As described in earlier chapters, clozapine was the first atypical antipsychotic developed and has some properties that set it apart from all of the other antipsychotics. Its side effect profile, as well as its efficacy profile, is quite different from both the typical and atypical antipsychotics, and it was largely considered the best development in treatment of schizophrenia since chlorpromazine. While it is not able to help everyone, or necessarily return people back to former functioning, it has been shown to be quite effective for use in treatment-resistant schizophrenia and therefore offers hope to many that they may get some relief from suffering. For this reason, it has been used throughout Europe for the past 30 years; however, it has only been used in the United States for about the past 20 years. One of the medication's other benefits is that it has a remarkably lower occurrence of movement side effects when compared to nearly all of the other antipsychotics. This is particularly relevant to patients with treatment-resistant schizophrenia. Patients with this disorder will require treatment with antipsychotics likely for decades. Most of the antipsychotics have the risk of causing tardive dyskinesia, a permanent movement disorder. Clozapine is unlikely to cause this side effect, which is another reason it can be a great option as treatment for this group of people. One of the other side effects of clozapine that makes it stand apart from other antipsychotics is the risk of a rare but dangerous blood disorder called agranulocytosis. The medication was actually first withdrawn from general use in the mid-1970s after deaths from this blood disorder were reported in Finland. Since then no other antipsychotics have been found to have the same properties leading to agranulocytosis. It is thought that this is because clozapine has a unique combination of mechanisms of action. The only other antipsychotic that has similar properties is olanzapine, which was created in an attempt to mimic clozapine in order to get its superior treatment effects. Olanzapine, however, has slightly different properties and fortunately does not have the side effect of the blood disorder but also unfortunately does not have the efficacy that clozapine has either.

Clozapine was taken off the market after deaths from agranulocytosis were reported; however, there was evidence from multiple different study cites showing that clozapine was more effective than the available antipsychotics, haloperidol or chlorpromazine. Although it had a life-threatening side effect, this seemed to be rare, and since it was found to be so effective in treating an illness that otherwise was not responding to medications, a pharmaceutical company remarketed the drug under controlled conditions in some European countries. In the United States, the FDA was not prepared to continue its use without further studies. The medication was off the market in the United States for about a decade, while research studies were done in order to prove to the FDA that the medication was demonstrably effective in its use for treatment-resistant schizophrenia. A study was completed and published that included patients with schizophrenia who had failed at least three adequate trials with antipsychotics and had not been in remission for at least five years. They compared clozapine with chlorpromazine and found that after taking the medication for four weeks, 2% of patients who took chlorpromazine showed improvement compared with about 33% of patients who took clozapine. It was then approved by the FDA; however, because of the risk of agranulocytosis, it was and continues to be marketed under a unique system requiring all patients taking the medication to be registered through a national registry that includes regular blood work to monitor for the development of the disorder.

For years there were multiple pharmaceutical companies that marketed clozapine, and each one of them had their own registry. The risk of agranulocytosis is higher when beginning the treatment with clozapine, so there are specific guidelines about how to monitor blood work throughout the use of clozapine. For the first six months of treatment with clozapine, a patient has to have a weekly blood test that monitors his or her white blood cell count. One of the first signs of agranulocytosis is a drop in white blood cell count. For the next six months of treatment it is required that they have blood work drawn every other week. After the first year of use, the monitoring is decreased to blood work drawn once a month and continues at that frequency for the time spent on the medication.

It used to be that each pharmaceutical company that marketed clozapine employed its own registry for monitoring. When a patient was started on the medication, the physician would register the patient with a specific registry. Each time that blood work needed to be reported, paperwork would be filled out monitoring the white blood cell count and sent to the specific registry. In 2015, there was an overhaul of the clozapine registry system, and the FDA announced that there would be changes made to the registry, monitoring, prescribing, dispensing, and receiving clozapine in attempts to address continuing safety concerns. There were two parts to the changes in these requirements. First, there was a clarification and enhancement of prescribing information further explaining how to monitor these patients. Second and more notably, the FDA approved a new shared registry to replace the existing registries maintained by the individual pharmaceutical companies. This new registry is called Clozapine REMS (risk evaluation and mitigation strategy) and was designed to help improve monitoring and management of patients with serious declines in white blood cell counts in response to clozapine treatment.

Clozapine REMS

One of the ideas behind the convergence of registries and emergence of one sole registry for the nation is that it is easier to monitor prescribing and lab work activity if it is all being input into the same place. So to begin the process, one of the first changes was that all prescribing providers and pharmacies needed to take a short test and register in the REMS system prior to being able to prescribe or dispense clozapine. The purpose of REMS is to use risk minimization strategies beyond the required drug labeling to ensure that the benefits of this medication outweigh the risks. The program has multiple goals, most centered around safety. They include educating prescribers, pharmacists, and patients about the risk of severe neutropenia and appropriate monitoring requirements, ensuring compliance with that monitor schedule before dispensing any medications, ensuring the prescriber documents a risk-benefit assessment if the patient has a drop in white blood cell count below an acceptable number, and establishing long-term safety and use of clozapine by enrolling all patients who receive it.

The risk of agranulocytosis is small but serious, so there have been multiple changes in regulations for monitoring and how to register patients for the medication over many years. In the United States, the FDA continues to work to make it as safe as possible while considering the sometimes incredible benefit the medication can have as well. The FDA continues to work to unify the regulation to ensure safe prescribing and use and seems to have gotten one step closer to that with the introduction of REMS. However, when you look at the use of clozapine throughout the world, the regulations are quite varied from region to region. One review paper looked at nine different countries to see how regulation of prescribing, dispensing, and monitoring of clozapine overlapped and differed (Nielsen et al. 2016). The review found that there was substantial variation in regulations and recommendations for clozapine use across the various regions starting with the most basic difference, formulation. All countries dispense an oral tablet, some also dispense an oral suspension, and others also dispense a disintegrating tablet. The Netherlands actually also has an injectable intramuscular form that is not available in other countries. The maximum daily dose is generally 900 mg/day in all of the countries except for one, Japan, where the medication is only licensed up to 600 mg/day. Even the indications for and approved usages for clozapine differ from country to country. In all countries it is approved for treatment-resistant schizophrenia, yet the definition of treatment-resistant is not a standardized term.

One thing that all countries have in common is a mandatory monitoring system for agranulocytosis. However, the system varies from country to country with some being stricter and others being slightly more lenient, and there have been no studies investigating the effects or prevalence of agranulocytosis based on different monitoring frequency. Some countries have a similar database to REMS that requires patients receiving clozapine to be registered and the pharmacies to double-check prior to prescribing in order to ensure that patients who had prior episodes of agranulocytosis or a decrease in white blood cells secondary to clozapine use are not exposed to the medication again. Other countries do not have a similar database. They still require the monitoring system to track blood work and prevent agranulocytosis but do not require input into a database prior to dispensing the medication. There is suggestion that the blood monitoring is reasonable for safety concerns, however, it makes the prescribing process more complex and may deter physicians from participating and using clozapine. Again, there are no studies that compare the different systems (database monitoring versus blood work monitoring alone) to determine whether they impact prescribing practices or safety profiles. One of the take-home messages from the review article is that clozapine is regulated differently in various parts of the world and that further research to determine which regulation systems are most appropriate in regard to safety, compliance, and cost-effectiveness is needed.

Clozapine is the most regulated antipsychotic and likely one of the most regulated medications prescribed in the United States. It has strict regulations because of its risk profile. Unfortunately, it is also one of the most effective antipsychotics and is likely underused. There are a number of reasons it is underused, but two of the main reasons are the concern about the side effect profile and the complexity of the regulation for prescribing and dispensing. The regular blood work monitoring and database registry are enough to deter patients and physicians from considering it as a potential treatment. While the regulatory systems are put in place for safety, they may end up decreasing use of the medication. More expansive studies of different implementation of monitoring systems would be beneficial in order to ensure creation of the most cost-effective, safe, and utilized clozapine regulation.

Clozapine has some of the most dangerous side effects and for that reason has federally mandated regulations, but as mentioned in previous chapters, all of the antipsychotics come with some risk of side effects. None of the other antipsychotics are federally regulated, however, many of them have guidelines for how to monitor for certain side effects over time, and many clinics implement their own guidelines and regulations to monitor for those. Each of the classes of antipsychotics has one main type of side effect that requires ongoing monitoring. For typical antipsychotics one of the most concerning side effects is movement disorders, notably tardive dyskinesia. While this is most prevalent in the typical antipsychotics, it can also be seen in the atypicals. One of the most concerning side effects when using atypical antipsychotics is the changes in the metabolic profile. For both of these classes of side effects there are clinical practice guidelines, and many clinics have instituted regulations in order to monitor and try to prevent these.

AIMS AND METABOLIC MONITORING

AIMS

The Abnormal Involuntary Movement Scale (AIMS) is a scale that was developed in order to monitor for changes in movement. As mentioned earlier, tardive dyskinesia is a movement disorder that is often incurable and is characterized by involuntary, repetitive body movements. It most commonly occurs as a result of long-term or high-dose antipsychotic use. For this reason, the AIMS was developed and used to monitor patients who are taking an antipsychotic. The scale is not meant to tell whether tardive dyskinesia is present or absent; it is only meant to observe the movements of the face, trunk, and limbs and rate them on a severity scale. The scale is generally given prior to starting an antipsychotic and should be administered annually while the person continues the antipsychotic. The scale will not tell you if the patient has the disorder or not, but it could guide clinical management. For example, if there were a younger patient taking a typical antipsychotic and after two years of treatment the AIMS began to show an increase in involuntary movements, the clinician would want to weigh the risks and benefits of trying a new medication, potentially leading to a decompensation of psychiatric symptoms versus continuing the medication, leading to an irreversible movement disorder. It seems that one would easily recognize these movement changes, and one could ask why a scale was necessary to monitor them. The changes in movement that lead to tardive dyskinesia generally begin subtly. It is during this early stage of changes that an intervention and switch to a medication which may have less likelihood to cause the disorder would be most beneficial. Therefore, the AIMS can be used to draw attention to the early changes and allow clinicians to make an early intervention that may be too late if not monitored regularly. Many mental health clinics have created their own system for regulation within the clinic to help guide clinicians and ensure that standards of care are being met. The AIMS only takes about 10 or 15 minutes to complete and can be done easily on a paper document or could be monitored via an electronic system. Many clinics require their clinicians to complete an AIMS yearly for all patients on an antipsychotic in order to maintain standards of care and follow practice guidelines.

Metabolic Monitoring

As mentioned earlier in the book, when discussing the side effects of antipsychotics, atypical antipsychotics commonly cause some changes in a patient's metabolic profile, meaning they can cause an increase in weight, body mass index (BMI), blood pressure, lipid levels, and blood sugar levels, which all have the potential to lead to further medical complications, including cardiovascular complications and diabetes. For this reason it is important to consider that risk when beginning the informed consent conversation with a patient who may benefit from an atypical antipsychotic. Again, there is no federal regulation to monitor for metabolic syndrome or any metabolic changes, however, it is prudent for clinicians to be monitoring some of these lab values when a patient is on an atypical in order to attempt to mitigate this risk and detect changes early so that they can be addressed, whether that means changing medications or treating the side effects. There have been many studies trying to determine the best practices for routine monitoring that target safety and effectiveness. However, different organizations may have different recommendations, and these recommendations have changed over the years and will likely continue to change with further developments in antipsychotics and further research. It is thought that these changes often occur when initiating the medication, so monitoring should occur more frequently for the first year. Clinicians should check a baseline weight, BMI, blood pressure, lipid panel, and hemoglobin A1C prior to starting an atypical antipsychotic so that there is an understanding of where the patient is at metabolically prior to starting the medication. Some people may already have elevated blood pressure or cholesterol or blood sugar prior to starting any medication. It would be important not only to understand what medical complications already exist because they may worsen but also to be able to tease out which changes might be secondary to the medication and which may be preexisting conditions. These values should then be followed throughout the treatment. There is no overarching regulatory agency monitoring this, but it is generally considered standard of care to check prior to starting and then check these values every three months for the first year of treatment. If the values are staying largely the same and are not trending up or concerning, then after a year of treatment and monitoring the frequency of monitoring could decrease to annual monitoring. Similarly to regulations in clinics with AIMS, many clinics have developed their own internal regulations to ensure that clinicians are keeping with standards of care and monitoring for metabolic syndrome regularly.

While there are few federally regulated antipsychotics at this time, it is possible that as more research is developed and management of health care continues to develop and change, monitoring practices for things like tardive dyskinesia and metabolic syndrome may become more regulated via either the state, insurance company, or federally.

In the grand scheme of things, antipsychotics are a relatively new and changing field of medications. Because of that they are not as well understood as some other classes of medications, and there is a lot of profit to be made from their use. Their production, distribution, and regulation are continuing to develop as more is understood about their benefits and risks and as more drugs come out onto the market. This has an impact on how they are viewed in society, by patients and by clinicians, which is an important aspect to be aware of and keep in mind when engaging in a conversation about them.

Chapter 8

The Social Dimensions of Antipsychotics

The extraordinary impact antipsychotics have had on society and health care is truly difficult to grasp. As much or more than any other class of medications, antipsychotics have allowed physicians to address illnesses that were long considered untreatable.

As discussed elsewhere in this text, antipsychotics are not perfect medications. In the first place, they do not cure illnesses; they treat illnesses by decreasing the intensity of symptoms. It would be fantastic if antipsychotics functioned like antibiotics, and patients suffering from mental illnesses could take medications for a course of 5 to 10 days and be completely free of the disease. Antipsychotics decrease the severity of the mental illness only during that time period when the patient is taking the medication. Antipsychotics also do not work with all patients. Some people with serious mental illnesses like schizophrenia are treatment-resistant, which means that for a variety of reasons, antipsychotics do not alleviate their symptoms, or, they may require an unusually large dose of antipsychotics. Further, antipsychotics have notable side effects. They cause sedation, movement disorders, metabolic complications, and other rare, but more serious adverse events.

However, despite the many flaws of antipsychotics, all mainstream mental health professionals agree that they are a tremendous improvement from the alternative treatments that preceded the medications. In fact, earlier treatments of the seriously mentally ill were so painful and dangerous that many families went to incredible lengths to keep their loved ones at home and shield them from medical professionals. They were often only taken to psychiatric hospitals when their symptoms or behaviors became so overwhelming or dangerous that the families had no other choice.

Therefore, the original major social impact of antipsychotics was that it allowed patients to be spared the traumatic, ineffective, and arguably inhumane treatments of mental illnesses that were in practice before chlorpromazine, the first antipsychotic, was introduced in the early 1950s. These included tooth removal, colectomy, cold-water baths, insulin-shock therapy, pyrotherapy, and lobotomies.

The second major social impact of antipsychotics was their ability to stabilize large numbers of patients and facilitate their discharge from large state hospitals that were widespread in this country at the dawn of the antipsychotic era. This transformation is called "deinstitutionalization," and the effects of this social phenomenon continue to be relevant in psychiatry today.

DEINSTITUTIONALIZATION

The state hospitals in the decades leading up to the 1950s and 1960s were massive institutions. The biggest ones housed thousands of patients and functioned essentially as independent cities. Pilgrim State Hospital in Suffolk County, Long Island, was the country's largest psychiatric facility and had about 14,000 patients at its peak census and employed several thousand more. The patients with serious mental illnesses that state hospitals discharged by the thousands needed somewhere to go. Psychiatrists realized that antipsychotics did not cure the illnesses but rather treated symptoms. Therefore, they needed mental health practitioners to continue to prescribe antipsychotics and monitor patients once they left the hospital. Doctors and politicians of the time also understood that the thousands of patients would need somewhere to live. The notion put forth by mental health professionals, in coordination with government administrators, was to transfer the treatment of the patients to outpatient providers in the community.

The first patients to leave the hospital were the most stable patients and the ones who had families that could support them and provide them housing. As the "deinstitutionalization" movement gathered steam, it became very popular and convenient for local and state governments. It was expensive to maintain thousands of patients in hospitals. Even though they were generally poorly staffed with nonideal living conditions, the state hospital system still employed thousands of workers and provided basic essentials for hundreds of thousands of patients. The shift of that economic burden to the families saved the government millions of dollars. Therefore, pressure grew to discharge as many patients as they could and even close down the hospital when possible.

Deinstitutionalization was, and continues to be, celebrated because it allowed patients with serious mental illnesses to retain more civil liberties. It allowed them to live freer lives, move as they pleased around the community, and have greater access to their family support systems. It also decreased the stigma of suffering from a serious mental illness because it did not automatically imply that the patient would be removed from their homes and locked up with other patients. However, deinstitutionalization had disadvantages, mostly for the patients.

Doctors quickly observed that treating patients in the community could be more difficult than treating them in the hospital. Good follow-up with a psychiatrist requires the patients to recognize that they have an illness, schedule appointments, remember the appointments, travel to the doctor's office, fill prescriptions, take medications several times per day, and be in good communication with the doctor if anything goes wrong. As described elsewhere in this text, one of the hallmark features of schizophrenia is delusions. Often, these delusions are grandiose in nature, leading patients to believe that they are powerful or invincible. Therefore, these patients are unlikely to accept the notion that they have a mental illness and need to take medications every day for the rest of their lives. Other classic features of schizophrenia are disorganized behavior, decreased motivation, paranoia, and isolative behavior. Given the nature of the illness, it is clear to see why a schizophrenic patient would be unlikely to use the newly established community mental health system appropriately. When the patients are in the hospital, it is much easier to facilitate compliance with medication and the necessary medical monitoring.

As a result, the revolving door phenomenon began. Too often, patients are stabilized in hospitals, discharged to the community, decompensate (become more symptomatic), and return to the hospital. Even though these patients are not in the hospitals permanently, they usually require more resources because their condition becomes acute.

Beyond requiring more resources, patients who frequently decompensate and have frequent hospitalizations have a worse prognosis than patients who are compliant with medications. To explain this concept another way, imagine two patients, Bert and Ernie, both 20 years old, who are impaired to the exact same degree by the same presentation of schizophrenia. Bert is always compliant with antipsychotics and therefore manages the illness reasonably well. As antipsychotics are not perfect medications, Bert still experiences some symptoms of paranoia, isolation, and disorganized behavior and speech. Every 5 or 10 years, Bert experiences a decompensation that involves acute psychosis, violent paranoid ideations, and crippling auditory hallucinations. These episodes are triggered by alcohol use, the loss of a loved one, or the occasional inability to access antipsychotic medication.

Ernie is less compliant with treatment. He rarely takes antipsychotics in the community and therefore suffers decompensations, involving the same acute symptoms as Bert, about every six months. When in the hospital, Ernie accepts medications and is able to be discharged to the community in three to four weeks. In 20 or 30 years, Bert will be much less impaired by schizophrenia than Ernie. Bert will have better cognitive functioning and better social skills and will show a better response to antipsychotics. Ernie will have more cognitive problems, will be less able to care for himself in the community, and will require higher doses of antipsychotics to treat delusions and hallucinations. The most commonly accepted hypothesis for the difference in the trajectories of these two patients is that psychotic episodes cause extensive damage to the brain. Therefore, because Ernie will have suffered more decompensations than Bert due to medication noncompliance, over the course of several decades, Ernie's brain will be more dysfunctional. Therefore, it can be argued that deinstitutionalization worsens the long-term prognosis for patients like Ernie. If Ernie stayed in an institution permanently, he would not suffer as many decompensations because doctors and nurses would help him take medications.

Another major problem with deinstitutionalization was, and continues to be, housing for the mentally ill. In the early phases, the patients who were discharged had families who could take them in. However, even patients who did not have stable housing or support in the community were eventually discharged as long as the antipsychotics were able to stabilize them in the hospital. This led to an enormous increase in the homeless population. Today it is common knowledge that homelessness is tightly correlated with serious mental illness. Studies vary, but approximately 70% of the homeless population in the United States has a serious mental illness such as schizophrenia, schizoaffective disorder, or bipolar disorder. However, prior to deinstitutionalization, a large portion of this population would have been patients in a state hospital.

Many psychiatric patients found even worse circumstances than homelessness. After deinstitutionalization, the percentage of the incarcerated population with a serious mental illness rose dramatically. This shift is intuitive and could have been predicted. There are many reasons why the mentally ill are at an increased risk of incarceration in prisons and jails. If a patient with schizophrenia is discharged from a hospital without proper housing, he or she may have great difficulty avoiding violations of minor local statutes against loitering or vagrancy. Further, given that disorganized behavior and speech are part of the diagnostic criteria for schizophrenia, it is easy to imagine how a patient with schizophrenia, especially if he or she is homeless, could frequently be found guilty of disturbing the peace or other "quality of life crimes." Next, given the disorganized behavior and other impairments that are seen with serious mental illnesses, it is logical that patients are not able to work consistently and are more vulnerable to poverty. Poverty in itself is a risk factor for crime because people come to the conclusion that it is necessary to steal in order to survive. Even if an impoverished person decides to ask for money instead of stealing it, panhandling too can be in violation of local laws that could lead to detainment by the police.

However, perhaps the most common crime the mentally ill commit, and therefore the most common reason they become incarcerated, is possession of illicit substances. There is a significant comorbidity of mental illness and substance use disorders. Commonly abused substances include marijuana, cocaine, crack cocaine, heroin, and newer synthetic substances like "K2" and "bath salts." Even though substances exacerbate the severity of the mental illnesses, people with serious mental illnesses are more likely to abuse them than the general population. Statistics vary depending on the exact study and the type of mental illness, but approximately 40–50% of people with a serious mental illness have a co-occurring substance use disorder, compared to about 10% of the general population. There are many explanations, but mental illness significantly detracts from a person's ability to "fit in" or feel good about himself or herself. Therefore, he or she is more likely to look for a quick way to feel better, even if that will make them feel worse in the long run.

Beginning in 1971, when Richard Nixon famously declared "war on drugs," the populations of jails and prisons have swelled. In 1980, there were approximately 500,000 people in prisons and jails. In 2014, there were over 2.3 million. Many of the prisoners were charged with low-level drug offenses, and many of them have serious mental illnesses.

However, much of the crimes committed by people with mental illnesses are driven by the same antisocial motivations as crimes committed by the general population. Due to a criminal's mental illness, it is possible that the crime would be poorly planned and executed, and the criminal would be more likely to be convicted than a criminal without a serious mental illness. Furthermore, people with mental illness, due to the high incidence of poverty, are less likely to be able to afford high-quality legal representation.

As a result of all of these factors, the population of people with mental illnesses in jails and prisons is enormous. About 15–20% of the country's incarcerated population has a serious mental illness, compared to about 2–4% of the general population. Prior to deinstitutionalization, many of these individuals would have been treated in state hospitals. However, after being discharged en masse by the state hospital system, many patients were unable to fully integrate in society and ended up in jails or prisons. Some critics of the deinstitutionalization movements consider it simply a shift of the mentally ill from hospitals, where they are treated, to jails, where they are punished. According to the National Alliance on Mental Illness (NAMI), 25–40% of people with mental illnesses will be incarcerated at some point of their lives. Currently, the country's largest "psychiatric hospitals," as defined as institutions treating the mentally ill, are the jails of the biggest cities in the United States, like Cook County Jail in Chicago and L.A. County Jail or Rikers Island in New York City. These corrections departments have the responsibility of treating thousands of patients who have needs that are much different than the rest of the inmates.

Another unfortunate outcome of deinstitutionalization was the decreased availability of long-term inpatient beds. Many of the state hospitals that discharged large numbers of patients closed because they were no longer needed. As a result, there are now relatively few spaces in hospitals for patients who need long-term care. After the decision is made that a psychiatric patient in an acute care facility requires a state hospital bed for long-term stabilization, he or she may have to wait months to find space.

The discussion above represents the negative consequences of deinstitutionalization. However, as mentioned previously, the newly found ability to leave the state hospital and live in the community, preferably with family, immensely improved the quality of life for many patients with serious mental illnesses. Patients who responded well to the earliest antipsychotics were able to work, spend time with families, and participate in community and religious activities. One type of psychotherapy, called logotherapy, focuses on helping patients find meaning in their lives. Logotherapy was developed by Viktor Frankl while working with victims of the Holocaust. Frankl, himself a Holocaust survivor, realized that happiness depended on our ability to find a purpose and direction in life. When patients are in hospitals for extended periods of time, they can feel as though their life has little meaning, and nothing they do matters. This feeling can lead to depression. It is easier to find important ways to spend time in the community. Therefore, as long as patients are able to find support in the community and maintain compliance with medication, deinstitutionalization allows patients to live more dignified and gratifying lives.

ANTIPSYCHOTICS AND THE DOCTOR-PATIENT RELATIONSHIP

Antipsychotics are similar to other classes of medication, in that they treat specific illnesses. However, there are unique aspects to antipsychotics that raise significant ethical and legal concerns. Antibiotics, for example, treat illness by targeting bacteria. They have essentially no effect on who we are as people or our identity. Antipsychotics also address medical conditions, like schizophrenia, but in this case, the illness is more a part of who the patient is. The illness deals with the process by which patients think, the specific thoughts they generate, and the things patients say. Therefore, to administer antipsychotics is, in a way, to change who a person is. Because this treatment is so central to a person's identity, the relationship between patient and psychiatrist must be open, based on trust and mutual respect.

A very common reason that patients stop taking antipsychotics, decompensate, and then require admission to a psychiatric facility is a disruption in the doctor-patient relationship. If patients are going to allow physicians to use their best judgment to prescribe medications that change who they are, they have to be very confident that the physicians know who they are and care deeply about their best interest. Mentally ill patients can have a keen awareness about the attitude of physicians. Even when patients are acutely psychotic and may have bizarre delusions or active auditory hallucinations, they are still capable of understanding that a psychiatrist is in a rush or if the psychiatrist is annoyed by the patient's disorganized behavior. They are very aware of the psychiatrists' bedside manner, and they may remember specific encounters with psychiatrists for years. Therefore, psychiatrists, more than any other physicians, must pay extremely careful attention to exactly how they act, what they say, and how they say it. No patient, no matter how psychotic they are, will take antipsychotics prescribed by doctors they do not trust.

Another reason physicians prescribing antipsychotics must develop a good rapport with patients is the fact that this class of medications has significant side effects. As discussed elsewhere in this text, side effects include sedation, sexual problems, weight gain, diabetes, hypertension, high cholesterol, and a host of movement disorders. Most patients would not tolerate these side effects and remain compliant with antipsychotics if they did not feel the physician was fully committed to their well-being. A grave mistake a psychiatrist can make is the failure to show patients that they are concerned with side effects. Sometimes, there is not much a doctor can do about side effects. However, they must listen thoroughly to patients and empathize with their struggles. If psychiatrists fail to show appropriate bedside manner, patients will not attend appointments and will not take the antipsychotics. As discussed earlier, noncompliance leads to more frequent decompensations, which implies a worse prognosis of the mental illness. Of course, even when a psychiatrist does not prescribe antipsychotics, the relationship between doctor and patient is important. Patients must trust doctors before they discuss their most difficult personal crises, like a troubled marriage or past trauma. However, due to their identity-altering nature, and particularly unpleasant side effects, antipsychotics have elevated the significance of the doctor-patient relationship.

Despite the fact that antipsychotics require a strong alliance, many psychiatrists are concerned about the distance antipsychotics and other psychiatric medicine put between doctor and patient. When the pharmaceutical industry developed pills that could address phenomena like depression and psychosis, many people spoke about the "medicalization" of mental illness. Essentially, this refers to the conception of a person's symptoms as a purely biological experience, like infection or inflammation. The reality is that the identification of biological bases of mental illness and the idea that a patient's personal history and psychological experience impact symptoms are not mutually exclusive. To truly understand someone's mental illness, the psychiatrist must understand both components.

No matter how biologically and technologically advanced the treatment of mental illness becomes, the reality is that psychological and social factors will always play an enormous role in a patient's outcome. It is necessary to understand how patients understand their illnesses. If they are ashamed or embarrassed to tell their family when they experience increased symptoms, like auditory hallucinations, they are less likely to reach out for the help they need. If there is a personal loss, like the dissolution of a marriage or the death of a loved one, a patient's symptoms are likely to worsen.

As discussed earlier, there is a large overlap between substance use disorder and serious mental illnesses. Therefore, psychiatrists must understand which substances their patients are abusing and the factors that lead to these dangerous behaviors. People with and without serious mental illnesses use substances like marijuana, alcohol, cocaine, and heroin for many different reasons. They can be self-medicating symptoms of mental illnesses, like depression or auditory hallucinations, when their prescribed medication has been ineffective. They could also use substances to address the side effects of the psychoactive medications. As mentioned previously, people with serious mental illnesses commonly use substances to forge relationships with others.

Further, how a patient spends his or her time has a critical impact on the trajectory of his or her mental illness. If a patient spends the entire day in bed or on the couch in front of the television, which is all too common, his or her life will lack the type of meaning Frankl discussed. He or she may then experience symptoms of depression. Patients, even those with intense and overwhelming symptoms, should keep themselves engaged with society in some form. Psychiatrists must understand how a patient lives to put his or her symptoms in context.

For the previous reasons, and many more, it is crucial for psychiatrists to look beyond the biological illness and treat the entire patient. Unfortunately, the "medicalization" of psychiatry that started with the development of antipsychotics and antidepressants has discouraged this robust and thorough approach. Largely due to economic forces, psychiatrists are often pressured to spend a decreased amount of time with patients, look only for specific symptoms, and prescribe corresponding medications, as if they are treating a purely biological disturbance, like strep throat.

This leads to poor mental health care. For example, imagine a 65-year-old woman who is prescribed antipsychotics for schizophrenia. During an appointment, the psychiatrist screens for symptoms of depression and finds that the patient, for the first time, describes symptoms that are consistent with a depressive episode. She reports feeling guilty, an inability to feel pleasure, depressed mood, difficulty sleeping, and fatigue. If the psychiatrist is purely focused on medicines and symptoms and only has 10 minutes for the session, he or she will start an antidepressant and see the patient again in several months. However, if a psychiatrist has the time and motivation to understand why the patient feels the way she does, he or she may find that the patient's only friend passed away and she is feeling more isolated than ever. Instead of prescribing an antidepressant, a more effective approach would be to empathetically listen to the patient's concerns and work with the patient to find her more support in the community, possibly at a community senior center or day program for people with mental illnesses.

Consider as well a 25-year-old male who is also treated with antipsychotics for schizophrenia. During an appointment, the psychiatrist asks about symptoms of psychosis. He or she realizes that the patient has increased auditory hallucination and is increasingly paranoid of his neighbors. If the psychiatrist is too narrow in his or her approach to treating mental illness, he or she may increase the dose of antipsychotics and see the patient in several months. However, if the physician had the time and a more holistic methodology, the patient might feel comfortable confiding in the doctor that he has been abusing cocaine recently, which exacerbates his psychotic symptoms. If the psychiatrist goes one step further to understand the patient's behavior, he or she may learn that the patient abuses cocaine because the antipsychotics are too strong and make him so sedated that he stays in bed the entire day. Cocaine is a stimulant and can increase energy but can also lead to cardiac problems, addiction, and incarceration. Therefore, the more appropriate direction over the long term would be to *decrease* as opposed to *increase* the dose of antipsychotics, so the patient is less sedated and does not require cocaine to function normally.

It is important to recognize that antipsychotics and other psychopharmacological agents have been critical in the fight against mental illnesses, allowing researchers to construct a biological mechanism for diseases. However, it is necessary for psychiatrists and mental health practitioners to retain perspective and to resist complete medicalization of these disorders and to resist any pressure to adopt a purely biological approach to treating patients. No matter how advanced and technical the field becomes, psychiatry will always be an art as opposed to a science.

LEGAL AND ETHICAL IMPLICATIONS OF ANTIPSYCHOTICS

Treatment over Objection

As discussed previously, antipsychotics change who we are, what we think, and what we say. As a result, this class of medication has the potential to be significantly controversial. One of the most legally and ethically difficult scenarios involves the administration of antipsychotics against the patient's will.

Patients are prescribed many types of medications against their will under specific conditions. For example, young children never accept vaccinations willingly; they are always forced by their parents to accept the shots. The reason nobody considers this a major ethical violation, other than the screaming toddler, is that parents know better than children. A small child does not understand the significance of illnesses like polio and measles, so they cannot properly weigh all the risks and benefits of vaccination. They would not, therefore, be capable of making proper medical decisions. The parents are capable, and common sense assigns them the responsibility of their children's medical decisions.

In medicine, this ability to make reasoned medical decisions is called capacity. While the example of toddlers lacking capacity to refuse vaccines is straightforward, many other capacity considerations are more difficult. For example, elderly patients have a hard time recovering from serious surgeries. About 50% of elderly patients become delirious in the hospital after hip replacements, which means that they may not know where they are, why they are in the hospital, or even who they are. If they are confused and decide to leave the hospital in the middle of the night against a doctor's recommendation, they could hurt themselves. If they do not understand what they are doing, they lack capacity, and the hospital staff has an ethical responsibility to keep them in the hospital against their will, just as a parent has an ethical responsibility to force a toddler to accept proper medical care. Another common reason patients may become delirious is infection. Bacterial infections of the central nervous system and other parts of the body like the urinary tract frequently have cognitive consequences and therefore compromise a patient's ability to render rational medical decisions. If patients have such an infection and because they are unable to fully appreciate the situation and they refuse treatment, doctors may give these patients antibiotics against their will.

What about psychotic patients who refuse to take antipsychotics? This is a frequently encountered situation because delusions are often part of the illnesses, so patients may be under false beliefs that obscure their ability to understand that they need these medications. The same standard, whether or not a patient has capacity to make medical decisions, is employed by physicians. However, there is a big difference between forcing someone to take antibiotics for a urinary tract infection and forcing someone to take antipsychotics to treat schizophrenia. As discussed previously, antipsychotics change who we are and how we think. The notion of forcing a patient to accept medications that change who they are presents a serious ethical dilemma. However, it is sometimes necessary for their safety and that of others in the community.

The matter of forcing patients to take antipsychotics is also legally complicated. The U.S. Constitution is very clear about the value of civil liberties. Many of the first 10 amendments to the Constitution, known as the Bill of Rights, deal with individual freedoms. Americans have the right to assemble, the freedom of religion, the freedom of speech, the freedom to a fair and public trial, and the freedom to own guns. The founding fathers were very wary of the establishment's intrusion on an individual's liberty. They were careful to state that the government is not allowed to quarter troops in someone's house, search people's property without just cause, or force people to testify against themselves in a trial. As a result, individual freedom is the core and essence of the American character. Americans take great pride in their ability to do whatever they want, as long as it does not directly infringe on someone else's rights. Possibly more than any other citizenry in the world, Americans value the right to be left alone by the government.

Perhaps the most relevant right granted by the First Amendment to the Constitution in this discussion is the freedom of expression. Generally, this clause involves political topics, like the right to burn the flag, but it also pertains to mental illness. Do not patients with schizophrenia have the right to express themselves, even if the majority of the population would label those expressions "crazy"? Antipsychotics change the way patients generate thoughts, the content of the thoughts, and the way patients speak. Is not, therefore, the forced administration of antipsychotics an enormous violation of the patient's freedom of expression, as guaranteed by the First Amendment to the Constitution of the United States?

The answer is yes, but it is more complicated. The government retains "police power" that authorizes the state to intervene when an individual poses a threat to himself or herself or others. Due to this delicate balance, many legal cases have been brought by patients and patient advocates. Individual states handle this complicated situation differently, based on the specific judicial decisions made by the highest courts in the respective states. The Supreme Court of the United States has not specifically ruled on this issue, and the Congress of the United States has not passed any specific legislation, so there is no unified policy throughout the country.

There are essentially two trends in how state governments regulate the forced administration of antipsychotics. One trend known as the "rights-driven approach" is used in many states, including Massachusetts and New York. This model emphasizes the individual civil rights of the patient. The Massachusetts policy was set by the district court case *Rogers v. Commissioner* (1983). Ruby Rogers was a woman who worked as a nurse's aide at Boston City Hospital when she was forced to stop working by symptoms of mental illness. She voluntarily admitted herself into a psychiatric hospital where she was prescribed antipsychotics. As she explained on the witness stand, the antipsychotics gave her intolerable side effects, so she refused to take them. When she refused, however, she testified that men would hold her down, force her to receive an injection, and leave her in a secluded room for a period of time. The court was sympathetic to Ms. Rogers's experience and established several guidelines. It said that whenever physicians want to administer medications over a patient's objection, a judge is required to confirm that the patient lacks capacity. Although, generally of a medical determination, the judges in this case decided that the administration of antipsychotics over a patient's objection is such a serious intervention that a judge's approval is required as a safeguard for the patient.

The other model is known as the "treatment-driven approach." This model emphasizes the delivery of treatment to patients who need it. New Jersey's treatment-driven approach is based on the case *Rennie v. Klein* (1983). John Rennie was a pilot and a flight instructor, described by many as highly intelligent. He developed symptoms of serious mental illness that included severe delusions. He was a "revolving door" patient; he was frequently stabilized in the hospital, discharged, stopped taking medication, and was readmitted. He frequently had delusions of being Jesus Christ, suicidal ideations, and the extremely worrisome symptom of stating that he wanted to kill President Gerald Ford. During his 12th hospitalization, he was given long-acting antipsychotic injections against his will, even though he was not acutely dangerous at the time. He sued the hospital, but the court ruled in favor of the hospital. The hospital at the time had a policy in place to protect the rights of the patient. If a patient disagreed with a physician and refused antipsychotics, there was an administrative review by more senior physicians. The court said that this review was sufficient and judges did not need to be involved in individual cases.

In all jurisdictions, emergencies are exceptions to the policies that govern treatment over objection proceedings. If hospital staff believes that a patient is an imminent risk to himself or herself or others, it can take action to medicate the patient. Further, it is important to understand how capacity applies to psychotic patients who refuse medications. Just being psychotic, which essentially means to disconnect with reality, is not a justification to treat a patient over his or her objection. The patient must lack the ability to make an informed decision. Therefore, if a patient understands that he or she has schizophrenia, and that antipsychotics would treat his or her symptoms, but he or she chose not to take them, perhaps due to the side effects, he or she will have that right under both of the models discussed previously. It is only when the patient is unable to appreciate that he or she has a mental illness or that the medications can help him or her, that he or she would lack capacity and therefore be treated over him or her objection.

There are other situations when the administration of antipsychotics has serious ethical and legal implications. It was decided by the U.S. Supreme Court in 1986 that insane prisoners cannot be executed. To do so would constitute cruel and unusual punishment, prohibited by the Eighth Amendment to the Constitution. If a prisoner on death row is insane, therefore, the state would have to wait until the patient regains his or her sanity, either naturally or with medications. However, what if a prisoner refuses medications? Does the state have a right to administer antipsychotics over the prisoner's objection just for the purpose of executing him or her? Such a case was brought before the Louisiana Supreme Court in the case *State v. Perry* (1992). Michael Owen Perry had a long history of schizophrenia and was convicted of murdering his parents, nephew, and two cousins. He was found to be incompetent to be executed, based on symptoms of his mental illness, and was treated with haloperidol over his objection. He sued that state, and the court upheld his claim. They wrote that even though he was on death row, he was still an American citizen and therefore had rights of privacy and was protected against cruel and unusual punishment. To force medications solely for the purpose of execution would have violated those protections. Haloperidol was discontinued, and the execution was indefinitely suspended.

In the late 1990s and early 2000s, lawmakers began to look for ways to mandate psychiatric treatment, usually in the form of antipsychotics, for certain patients in the community as opposed to only patients in the hospital. The essential premise was that many patients habitually refuse to take medications outside of the hospital. The most common reason patients stop taking medications are the unpleasant side effects, an inability to recognize that they need medications, or the lack of organization necessary to attend appointments and take medications consistently. When some of these patients are noncompliant in the community, their symptoms, including paranoia, agitation, and disorganization, represent serious threats to the community. When they are hospitalized and given antipsychotics either voluntarily or involuntarily, they no longer are dangerous, and, therefore, psychiatrists have no legal authority to retain them in the hospital. However, their discharge remains a danger due to the pattern of noncompliance.

In 1999, this hypothetical scenario was realized and resulted in tragedy. Andrew Goldstein was a 29-year-old man with a known history of schizophrenia and was frequently noncompliant with antipsychotics in the community. After becoming agitated on a subway platform in New York City, Goldstein pushed Kendra Webdale in front of an oncoming train, resulting in her death. Local legislators, working closely with Kendra's family, developed Kendra's Law, signed by Governor George Pataki in 1999.

Kendra's Law established the criteria of assisted outpatient treatment (AOT). As of 2015, 44 states and many other countries and localities have adopted similar laws. In each jurisdiction, the details of AOT, also known as "outpatient commitment," differ, but the principles are consistent. In New York State's AOT program, a patient is required to maintain compliance with a certain treatment plan. This may include any combination of medications, drug screening, and appointments with mental health professionals. If a patient is in violation of the terms of the outpatient commitment, the police or emergency medical services (EMS) have the authority to bring patients against their will to a hospital, where they can be evaluated for up to 72 hours. Normally, if a person does not exhibit any symptoms that could be interpreted as a danger to himself or herself or others, police or EMS would not be legally justified in taking him or her anywhere without consent. However, AOT authorizes them to do just that. If, due to noncompliance with medication, staff at the hospital does indeed find the patient to be an acute danger to himself or herself or others, he or she would be committed to the hospital, where he or she could receive involuntary medications by the processes described previously. If the patient is not found to be acutely dangerous to himself or herself or others, he or she would be discharged to the community. However, as long as the patient is in violation of the terms of the AOT order, he or she can be brought to the hospital by authorities at any time. Needless to say, this is an unpleasant experience for patients, which serves as a motivation to comply with the mandated outpatient treatment.

The physicians and legal authorities that developed and continue to manage AOT understood that to prevent relapse of serious mental illnesses, a robust treatment plan is necessary. Therefore, to "commit" a patient to AOT, the psychiatrist must submit a treatment plan that usually consists of which medications a patient must take, where the patient would live, where he or she would receive psychiatric care, and what, if any, substance abuse program he or she would attend. All components of AOT must be met in order for a patient to remain compliant with the program. Therefore, even if a patient is attending appointments and taking medications, if he or she does not live where they are stipulated to live, he or she can be found in violation of AOT and brought to the emergency room for an evaluation. The rationale for this component of AOT is that patients with serious mental illnesses often require stable, consistent environments to comply with medications, attend appointments, and avoid substances. The treatment plan should mandate that the patient remain in the most supportive environment possible. Therefore, if anything changes in the patient's environment, the AOT coordinators want to respond before the change leads to a potentially violent decompensation. The mission of AOT after all is to prevent the type of tragedy that led to Ms. Webdale's death.

Because outpatient commitment is a significant infringement on a citizen's freedom, many jurisdictions, including New York, require a judge's approval. Even when patients agree to AOT because they believe it will be in their best interest, judges are still required to grant the order.

Only certain patients are eligible for outpatient commitment. In New York, the criteria, as stipulated by Kendra's Law, are summarized next:

- Patients must be 18 years old or older.
- Patients must have a diagnosed mental illness.
- Patients must be unlikely to survive safely in the community without supervision.
- Patients must have been hospitalized at least twice due to lack of compliance with treatment for mental illness within the past 36 months.
- Patients must have demonstrated serious violent behavior toward themselves or others within the past 48 months.
- Patients must be unlikely to voluntarily participate in treatment.
- Patients must be likely to benefit from AOT.

A significant amount of research has been devoted to understand the results of the implementation of AOT program. Studies have yielded mixed results, but the generally accepted opinion is that increased resources and supervision allow patients with mental illnesses to remain in the community safely for longer periods of time.

The treatment plans for AOT patients invariably include antipsychotics, because almost all patients referred for AOT suffer from a psychotic illness. However, due to the context of the patient's treatment, the medications are specifically chosen to improve compliance. Patients are only assigned to AOT when they are unable to remain compliant with medications in the community. As discussed elsewhere in this text, antipsychotics are available in several formulations. They are mostly prescribed in pill form, to be taken orally. However, they can be given intravenously to medically hospitalized patients or as an injection. Injectable antipsychotics can be fast-acting, in cases of emergencies, or long-acting. Long-acting antipsychotics, given every two to four weeks, have the advantage of not requiring patients to remember to take medications every day. Long-acting injectable antipsychotics have been shown to improve compliance with medications. Usually, patients on AOT will have treatment plans that specifically call for long-acting antipsychotic injections, due to previous incidence of noncompliance.

ANTIPSYCHOTICS AND POLITICAL DISSENT

The ability of individuals to deem a patient "mentally ill" and commit them to a hospital is a potentially dangerous responsibility. Citizens who are jailed after committing crimes are entitled the safeguards of the criminal justice system, including a trial, a jury, and so on. However, patients who are committed to a psychiatric hospital have fewer protections, depending on the jurisdiction. At least in the short term, it only requires several doctors to decide that hospitalization is warranted. As a result, the process of forcing people into psychiatric institutions carries the potential for serious abuse. Several authoritarian government regimes have used mental illness as a pretext to remove inconvenient citizens from the community, embarrass them, or coerce them to retract positions that criticize the government.

Authorities in the Soviet Union infamously labeled dissents as mentally ill. A "diagnosis" they often used was "anti-Soviet agitation." An investigation by several world bodies found that some critics of the Soviet government were found not responsible of their crimes due to "medical reasons." They were then taken to hospitals and given antipsychotics against their will. The physicians in these cases were treating patients' "delusions of reformism" and "anti-Soviet thoughts." Further, it was revealed in interviews that some "patients" were administered high-dose antipsychotics as a punishment for breaking certain prison/hospital rules.

In 2010, a series of articles in the *New York Times* exposed similar abuses by the Chinese government. One article described the case of Xu Lindong who filed several complaints against the local government regarding a land dispute. He was confined for over six years in psychiatric hospitals and was routinely forced to take antipsychotic medications, despite the absence of any identifiable mental illness. The main problems identified were a lack of mental health law that appropriately protected patients and psychiatrists who were vulnerable to pressure by government officials. It was also rumored that Chinese government officials imprisoned members of the spiritual group Falun Gong in psychiatric hospitals under the pretext of treating mental illnesses.

During the military Junta in Uruguay in the 1970s, psychiatrists working with the military regime were accused of many ethical violations. They repeatedly broke patients' confidentiality and provided often damaging information to the military commanders. They were also accused of administering antipsychotics at high doses with the aim of inducing painful side effects.

Psychiatrists, and all physicians, must maintain their sole duty to their patient and only act in his or her best interest. In addition to the example given previously, physicians have in recent history practiced medicine in a way that has greatly abused their patients. The core problem generally surrounds this issue of duty. Physicians who have been complicit in this type of patient abuse typically practice medicine with a duty to either the government or some perceived greater public good. Doctors must consider only the patient with very few exceptions, including situations when a patient has a dangerous contagious disease, like Ebola virus, or the patient discusses plans to kill somebody. In those cases, doctors have ethical and legal obligations to consider other people beside the patient in their actions. Otherwise, a physician's only responsibility is to the patient.

ANTIPSYCHOTICS AND THE ELDERLY

One area of specific concern among many mental health practitioners and advocates for senior citizens is the use of antipsychotics in the geriatric population. Elderly patients are especially vulnerable to the side effects of antipsychotics. They are more likely to experience dizziness, falls, and cardiac problems than adults. Further, antipsychotics have a specific "black box warning" with use in the elderly, which is essentially a warning to physicians that a medication can have serious side effects. In this case, elderly patients who take antipsychotics have been shown having an increased risk of death, from a wide range of conditions, when compared to other adult patients.

Despite these concerns, antipsychotic use is extremely common in nursing homes and in geriatric populations in other settings. Many patients with dementia exhibit behavioral problems. It is less common that patients with dementia have psychosis, but it is frequently seen. It is extremely difficult to care for dementia patients, especially when their behavior includes punching, kicking, spitting, and screaming. These behaviors can be addressed with certain behavioral interventions, like reminding dementia patients where they are, speaking to them in a reassuring tone of voice, and engaging them on topics that were of interest to them in their pre-dementia lives. Caregivers frequently experience "burnout" and can develop symptoms of anxiety and depression themselves. Therefore, it is very common for caregivers to give elderly patients antipsychotics as a way to calm them down, even if they do not have any psychotic symptoms. A caregiver, like a home health aide, or a nurse at a nursing home, may give an elderly patient antipsychotics after minimal behavioral symptoms so they can have a more relaxing shift.

Currently, approximately 300,000 nursing home residents in the United States are prescribed antipsychotics. Most of these residents are not prescribed antipsychotics for indications approved by the Food and Drug Administration (FDA), like bipolar disorder or schizophrenia. Rather, they are given for symptoms associated with dementia like agitation and frustration. When patients are prescribed medications for reasons that are not specifically cited by the FDA, it is called "off-label" use. Off-label use of any medication is inherently more risky because it is not supported by as much data, and a favorable benefit to risk ratio has not been established by the FDA. In March 2012, the federal government launched an initiative to decrease the number of off-label prescriptions given in nursing homes by 15% by December of that year. The goal was met, but not until September 2014. However, antipsychotic use in the elderly is decreasing.

ANTIPSYCHOTICS AND CHILDREN

Other than the elderly, another historically vulnerable population with worrisome antipsychotic use has been children. The trend of prescribing antipsychotics in nursing homes to address agitation in the elderly mirrors the use of antipsychotics in children to treat behavioral problems.

Psychosis is rare in children and adolescents. Psychotic disorders like schizophrenia or schizoaffective disorder typically emerge in late adolescence or early adulthood. Psychiatrists are often consulted when children describe visual and auditory hallucinations, especially when there are accompanying behavioral problems. However, those descriptions are much more likely to be products of typical childhood imagination than genuine psychosis.

Antipsychotics are also effective in treating mania associated with bipolar disorder. Bipolar disorder also typically presents in early adulthood. When it is diagnosed in children or early adolescents, it is typically based on mood swings, behavioral problems, and irritability. Therefore, the role of antipsychotics in patients with the diagnosis of bipolar disorder, but who do not have mania at the time of treatment, and have never had a clear manic episode, is not well defined.

Although uncommon, psychosis can occur in early adolescence and childhood, sometimes in children as young as five years old. This is typically seen when children have a strong family history of a psychotic disorder, such as a child whose parents suffer from schizophrenia. In these rare cases, antipsychotics are necessary and effective.

Nonetheless, antipsychotics are prescribed widely to children in the United States. They are prescribed to many children who suffer from clear psychosis or mania. The FDA has approved certain antipsychotics for other uses. One of the most commonly utilized is the indication to treat irritability associated with autism in children as young as five (risperidone) and six (aripiprazole). However, many children are prescribed antipsychotics to control concerning behaviors that occur in the absence of diagnoses like autism, bipolar disorder, or schizophrenia. In fact, 63% of children treated with antipsychotics have diagnoses that describe behavioral problems, as opposed to one of the aforementioned indicated diagnoses.

The administration of antipsychotics to children involves several specific concerns. Chief among them is the notion that the human brain develops well into the 20s. Individual cells throughout the brain, specifically the frontal cortex, which is responsible for planning and decision making, are reinforced through a process called myelinization. This involves the neuron's insulation in a sheath of a fatty substance called myelin. This process makes the cell more effective. Therefore, many of the psychiatric illnesses or behavioral problems seen in children may resolve naturally after the brain matures. Medicating children may alter the natural development of the brain or obscure parents' and physicians' ability to understand if ameliorated symptoms are attributable to antipsychotics or personal maturation. Further, researchers are not aware of the long-term effects of antipsychotics started in childhood, because these prescribing practices are relatively new. It is impossible to say what the risks are for a five-year-old started on risperidone when they are 65, because no 65-year-old today has taken risperidone since they were five—it did not exist then. Other antipsychotics did exist 60 years ago, specifically chlorpromazine, but it was not prescribed to five-year-olds.

Another major concern is the metabolic side effect profile of the second-generation antipsychotics, which is the class overwhelmingly prescribed to children and adolescents. Childhood obesity is at a major national crisis point.

Childhood obesity has a negative impact on a child's self-esteem and physical health.

In the United States in 2010, children aged six and younger were given 270,000 prescriptions for antipsychotics. Children aged 7–12 were given 2.14 million antipsychotics prescriptions. Adolescents were prescribed more antipsychotics than any other age groups. Approximately 2.8 million prescriptions were distributed to patients between the ages of 13 and 18. The frequency of prescribing antipsychotics to children and adolescents increased dramatically between the late 1990s and early 2000s. Since then, the rate has roughly leveled off.

Due to the concerns of prescribing antipsychotics to children, young patients should be treated by psychiatrists with training in child and adolescent psychiatry. Psychiatrists who choose to specialize in treating younger patients complete a two-year training program after completion of general psychiatric training. Unfortunately, there are not enough child and adolescent psychiatrists to treat all the children who are prescribed antipsychotics. As a result, only about 30–40% of patients aged 18 and younger, who are prescribed antipsychotics, are seen by psychiatrists with specialized expertise.

WHEN TO TREAT? THE IMPLICATIONS OF THE INITIATION OF ANTIPSYCHOTIC TREATMENT

The decision to initiate antipsychotic treatment has significant medical and ethical implications. Theories differ in the optimal timing of starting treatment for the first time. When looking at psychotic illness from a purely medical model, it would be most appropriate to start treatment as soon as symptoms are present. There would be no reason to delay giving a patient antibiotics for an infection. To do so would put the patient at risk of more severe illness. Why wait to give a patient antipsychotics after a psychiatrist identifies symptoms of psychosis?

Although research into illnesses like schizophrenia has advanced our understanding significantly, there is much about psychotic illness that remains unknown. Also, mental illness is a more individual, idiosyncratic process than infection. The cause underlying one person's psychosis may be completely different for someone else.

It is conceivable that some psychoses may resolve naturally or never reach the severity that requires long-term antipsychotic use. At times, people who are in significant emotional distress may undergo a brief psychotic reaction that can include paranoia or auditory hallucinations. These patients may be better off without antipsychotics.

A significant debate in psychiatry revolves around the timing of starting antipsychotics for adolescents with new-onset psychotic illness, like schizophrenia. The typical presentation of schizophrenia, discussed elsewhere in the text, involves a prodromal period. Essentially this is a period of several months when the patient becomes more withdrawn and less communicative than normal. His or her grades in school and relationships with friends will likely suffer. After the prodromal period, more classic signs of schizophrenia, like delusions and hallucinations, emerge. Generally, psychiatrists wait until the onset of these symptoms to prescribe antipsychotics. However, data have shown that early identification and treatment lead to an improved outcome. Psychiatrists may delay treatment due to a shared sense of denial with the patient and the family. The diagnosis of a young person with a serious mental illness is a devastating experience for a family, and psychiatrists are understandably reluctant to do so. However, deferring this difficult responsibility may only serve to delay necessary treatment.

THE BUSINESS OF ANTIPSYCHOTICS

It is impossible to discuss the social dimensions of antipsychotics without appreciating the fact that they have become a billion-dollar industry. This topic is further developed elsewhere in this text, but the notable social implications of the pharmaceutical industry require a brief discussion in this chapter.

During the period between July 2011 and June 2012, Abilify (aripiprazole) was the most valuable antipsychotic for the pharmaceutical industry and generated $5,434,400,000 in revenue. Seroquel (quetiapine) came in second at $3,672,400,000. Zyprexa (olanzapine) and Geodon (ziprasidone) each grossed more than a billion dollars during that time period. Antipsychotics as a whole represented a $20.8 billion industry in 2011. The profit margins have decreased slightly since then overall, but antipsychotics remain an engine in the pharmaceutical industry. In the 12 months leading up to March 2014, Abilify was not just the most profitable antipsychotic, it was the highest grossing medication overall, netting $6.9 billion for Otsuka Pharmaceutical.

Whenever incredibly large profits are accessible, the pharmaceutical firms that develop and manufacture antipsychotics will compete to capture as big of a share of that market as possible. Companies have attempted to sell their product by making the drugs seem appealing by downplaying, or worse, hiding the potential side effects from patients and physicians. In 2012, a judge in Arkansas ordered the pharmaceutical company Johnson and Johnson to pay $1.2 billion in fines over their deceptions in marketing Risperdal (risperidone), by minimizing side effects including weight gain, diabetes, and strokes.

In 2009, the pharmaceutical giant Eli Lilly was forced to pay nearly $1.5 billion for manipulative advertising of Zyprexa (olanzapine). Pharmaceutical companies are not allowed by law to advertise their product for any indication that does not have specific FDA approval. Physicians are allowed to prescribe medications off-label, but, of course, by practicing medicine that is not grounded in robust evidence, they are more vulnerable to malpractice lawsuits. According to the government, Eli Lilly marketed their product as a treatment for dementia. The lawsuit, which included criminal complaints, alleged that the company printed product information and trained their drug representatives to instruct physicians that Zyprexa was effective for managing agitation associated with dementia.

MENTAL ILLNESS AND VIOLENCE

Mental health has taken on a new sense of national urgency in recent years due to several high-profile violent acts committed by individuals with mental illnesses. There has been significant debate about accessibility of mental health resources in the community, the adequacy of supervision of patients with histories of violence, the availability of guns to individuals with mental illness, and patients' compliance with medications.

This is a complicated and controversial subject. Although there have been several crimes carried out by patients with mental illnesses, there have been many myths circulated in the public about the connection between mental illness and violence. Many people assume people with serious mental illnesses are significantly dangerous. The reality is that only about 3–5% of violent crimes are committed by individuals with illnesses such as schizophrenia. That is somewhat higher than the percentage of the population with serious mental illnesses, implying a correlation between the illness and violence. However, certain media coverage and dialogue in the general public may give the impression that people with mental illnesses are responsible for a large majority of violence in this country, which is categorically false. Substance use disorders, which are much more prevalent and arguably less stigmatized than psychotic disorders, lead to significantly more violence. In fact, people who suffer from serious mental illnesses are much more likely to be the victims of violent crimes than the perpetrators.

Furthermore, when patients with serious mental illnesses commit violent crimes, it is often not the psychosis that drives the crimes, but rather the same factors that drive violence committed by individuals without mental illnesses. These include poverty, substance use, antisocial and narcissistic personality disorders, and impulsivity. Psychosis often manifests as intense paranoia. Patients with active symptoms of schizophrenia are therefore more likely to attempt to avoid interactions with others at all costs, even if it leads to their inability to secure consistent food and shelter. The typical counterexample to that trend is when a patient's paranoia becomes acute and specifically involves another individual. The patient may come to the false conclusion that he or she is acting in self-defense, leading to violence.

There have been several mass shootings in the country in recent history that continue to resonate with the public. Attacks at Newtown, Connecticut, Virginia Tech University, San Bernardino, California, and Littleton, Colorado, are ingrained on our national consciousness. While anyone who kills innocent people could qualify for a mental illness, such as a personality or mood disorder, it was not clear that any of the respective assailants had a primary psychotic disorder such as schizophrenia or schizoaffective disorder. However, other catastrophes at Tucson, Arizona, Washington, DC, and Aurora, Colorado, did involve individuals with psychotic disorders, and, therefore, antipsychotics play a role in this debate. When patients are compliant with medications, they are significantly less likely to engage in violence borne out of paranoia or disorganized thoughts.

On January 8, 2011, Jared Lee Loughner gathered a small arsenal and attempted to assassinate U.S. Representative Gabrielle Giffords. In the process, he killed six people, included a federal judge. Until his mass murder, his descent from stability into psychosis does not appear atypical. Acquaintances explained that Loughner was a likable person and a good friend until his personality changed in adolescence. His behavior became bizarre, unpredictable, and disconnected from other people. He then became paranoid and was consumed by conspiracy theories. This spiraled into a hatred of politicians and his eventual crime. Although he was found to be responsible for his actions (as opposed to not guilty by reason of insanity), Loughner was diagnosed with schizophrenia and has been treated with antipsychotics in prison. It is likely that if there were more awareness of mental illness with less stigmatization, Loughner could have been treated prior to the crime, preventing the destruction of so many lives and communities.

About 18 months later, with the country still recovering, James Holmes opened fire on a movie theatre in Aurora, Colorado, during a screening of the Batman movie, *The Dark Knight Rises*. Holmes had seen several mental health professionals at the college he briefly attended, but he did not continue to receive sufficient services in the community after he was no longer a student. He planned the attack extensively, including planting explosives in his apartment to target police after the crime. He was also found responsible, although he entered a plea of not guilty by reason of insanity. He was given different diagnoses by court-appointed psychiatrists who interviewed him after the attack, including schizotypal personality disorder and schizoaffective disorder. However, he was found sane, responsible for his actions, and sentenced to life in prison.

The most infamous crime that involved mental illness, before the recent series of mass shootings, took place on March 30, 1981. John Hinckley Jr. attempted to assassinate then-President Ronald Reagan. He seriously injured several people, including President Reagan, when a bullet ricocheted of the presidential limousine and hit him in the chest. Hinckley was diagnosed with schizophrenia by the defense's expert psychiatrist, and he was found not guilty by reason of insanity. Therefore, instead of prison, Hinckley was transferred to a secure psychiatric facility, St. Elizabeth's Hospital, in Washington, DC. Other than involving a president, the Hinckley case was unusual due to the nature of the attack. Hinckley had developed an obsession with the movie star Jodie Foster and planned to get her attention by committing this violent act. Hinckley's deteriorating condition was known to his family, who attempted to get him evaluated and treated. He was not in consistent treatment and was not taking antipsychotics at the time of the attack.

In the public debate over violence and mental illness, significant attention is given to the availability of mental health resources. This is an important topic. Many people have to wait months to see a mental health professional, and some are unable to afford proper care. However, in the cases described previously, and in the vast majority of cases when mental illness and violence intersect, the problem is not access to care. All three assailants described previously could have, and at times did, received attention of mental health professionals. The problems were the individuals' lack of insight into their illness and the limited ability of onlookers to intervene. As mentioned earlier, the best way for society to address this problem in the future is to decrease the stigma of mental illness and the use of antipsychotics under the direction of a psychiatrist. If the suggestion of a friend to see a mental health professional and start medications were perceived as nonjudgmental, like a suggestion to take antibiotics for strep throat, it would be easier to help people treat their mental illnesses. However, if taking antipsychotics is associated with the connotation of being "crazy" or dangerous, patients will be in denial of their mental illnesses and avoid treatment as long as possible. This will lead to more serious illness, more suffering for the patient, and likely more cases of violent acts.

Chapter 9

The Future of Antipsychotics

Thus far this book has covered a lot of information about antipsychotics in an attempt to create a well-rounded understanding of the class of medications. It has started with the history, exploring how the medications were originally discovered and further developed. It looked at the various different disorders that the medications have been used to treat. It worked to explain how the class of medications works as a whole and some of the differences in the mechanisms of action in the individual medications as well as the risks of side effects. Prescription medications are often understood in the medical field and viewed by the general population in some type of vacuum, without considering the larger social context. This book has attempted to include that social context in order to create a more open and well-rounded understanding and conversation about the medications. It has been discussed and stated many times previously that antipsychotics are not perfect medications. They have, however, provided many people suffering with chronic, debilitating diseases with some relief. This, of course, is a simplistic understanding of the medications, and the book in general has worked to help create a deeper and more complete understanding of risks and benefits and clinical and social implications of the use of antipsychotics. The next step is to take a look at the class of medications and where they are going from here. To understand where the medications might be going next, where their future may lay, it is prudent to first look at where they are currently failing. If there is a good understanding of where the medications are falling short, then there is a clear direction for new research and development. There are currently newer drugs that are under research and new formulations of medications that may improve clinical response, which will also be discussed.

WHERE ARE ANTIPSYCHOTICS FAILING?

Earlier in the book there was focus and discussion about the effects and applications of antipsychotics. The focus in that chapter was on antipsychotics' effectiveness in treating psychotic symptoms, most notably positive psychotic symptoms. Recall from earlier that positive psychotic symptoms can be thought of as the psychotic symptoms that are most notable by the outside population. Take for example, a person is seen on the street clearly talking out loud, as if he were having a conversation, but no one else is around. This person is likely responding to auditory hallucinations, a positive psychotic symptom. Or, a person who appears a bit bizarre, dressed in eccentric clothing, and when you speak with him or her, you cannot follow the conversation because the speech pattern is disorganized; this is a thought disorder, another positive symptom. These are just two examples of positive psychotic symptoms that can be easily identified by a stranger, someone not familiar with the person's mental illness. As discussed earlier, the positive psychotic symptoms are generally at least somewhat responsive to antipsychotic treatment.

On the other hand, negative psychotic symptoms are historically extremely difficult to target and treat. As mentioned earlier in the book, the negative symptoms are the psychotic symptoms that are not as easy to identify from an outside perspective. The negative symptoms are more related to a person's emotions, cognitions, and motivations. Those suffering with negative symptoms will often appear to not show any emotion, will lack pleasure or interest in activities, will often have no motivation to do daily activities, and will have some cognitive slowing. While the positive psychotic symptoms can be quite disruptive, the consensus is that the negative psychotic symptoms, especially because they are so difficult to treat, have the greatest detrimental impact on a person's long-term level of functioning. Initially this can be difficult to understand as it seems that the more noticeable symptoms would likely cause the most distress and impairment. Psychotic symptoms are prevalent in schizophrenia, which is a disorder that usually starts in young adulthood. The positive symptoms can often be treated with antipsychotics but the negative symptoms often linger and lead to prolonged impairment. The estimates for the cost of treatment and loss in productivity associated with schizophrenia are upward of $60 billion annually. The majority of those costs, at least three quarters, are thought to be secondary to loss in productivity as opposed to the actual cost of treatment. This loss of productivity is usually secondary to ongoing negative psychotic symptoms. People with ongoing negative symptoms struggle with many functional impairments and often require some type of public assistance, and the large majority are unable to sustain employment and rely on others for financial support. Research suggests that improvement in negative symptoms is associated with multiple improved functional outcomes, including social functioning and independent living skills. For a number of years, treatment of negative symptoms has been identified as a critical area of treatment with unmet needs thus far, making research and development of antipsychotics that would target and treat negative symptoms more effectively a high priority.

As discussed earlier in the book, part of the goals behind developing the atypical antipsychotics was to develop medications that would be more effective in treating the negative symptoms of psychosis while reducing other movement side effects at the same time. Clozapine, which is the first atypical developed, has actually been shown to do both of those things. It is effective in reducing both positive and negative symptoms and has a lower occurrence of extrapyramidal side effects. Unfortunately, clozapine has a risky side effect profile, so other atypical antipsychotics were developed. Each atypical developed was with the hope that it would be a newer, better, and more effective antipsychotic. There are some specific areas where the atypical antipsychotics differ from each other, but generally speaking, other than clozapine, they have similar efficacy profiles and have not been found to be very effective in targeting negative symptoms.

Another area of treatment where antipsychotics are at least struggling, perhaps failing, is in the treatment of resistant psychosis. Throughout this book, we have discussed clozapine fairly extensively as it stands out from the other antipsychotics. It has been shown to be more effective than the other antipsychotics in treatment-resistant psychosis. However, we have shown that it is often underutilized, has a risky side effect profile, has a demanding blood work monitoring schedule, and is sometimes not tolerated by patients. Additionally, while clozapine is more effective than other antipsychotics in treatment-resistant schizophrenia, it still has much room for improvement. Guidelines suggest that clozapine can and should be initiated after someone fails two trials of treatment with different antipsychotics. However, even with initiation of clozapine following those guidelines, up to 40% of patients have only partial remission and even more do not reach a full level of functional recovery. For all of those reasons there has been a push to develop more medications, similar to clozapine, that would be more effective in the treatment.

Current practice, in order to address both negative symptoms and treatment-resistant psychosis, generally leads to polypharmacy, with multiple medications in the same class and/or augmentation with medications from other classes. Clinicians will add on second or third antipsychotics in order to try target symptoms that have been resistant. They will also add on medications in other classes like mood stabilizers or antidepressants, with the hope of decreasing some symptoms that the single antipsychotic is unable to. Reviews of patients with schizophrenia on polypharmacy have shown conflicting information regarding the efficacy of polypharmacy and its impact on mortality rates. There is some information out there to suggest that there is some benefit to adding a second atypical antipsychotic to clozapine if there is only partial response. There is also some evidence to suggest that adding an antidepressant to an antipsychotic for patients with negative symptoms may provide some benefit. There is little to no evidence for any specific medication augmentation to address the cognitive dysfunction that occurs with schizophrenia. Still, all of this requires further research with larger randomized controlled studies in order to make clear recommendations. And even with further studies, the consensus has and continues to be that the available medications are not enough. There is an ongoing push for more exploration of the molecular neurobiology of psychosis which would hopefully lead to novel treatments that can target some of the areas that current antipsychotics are not addressing well, specifically negative symptoms, cognitive deficits, and treatment-resistant psychosis.

One of the more challenging aspects when discussing the current state or future progression in the field of antipsychotics is the fact that the field is pushing for advancement and so develops many new medications over a relatively short period of time or in bursts. There is a strong desire on the part of researchers and clinicians as well as patients to have more successful medications, which may cloud or influence initial responses to new medications. Also, although there is research done prior to the approval of and release of medications to the market, it takes time once a medication is on the market to study its true effectiveness and likelihood of side effects. The direction since the development of the class of second-generation antipsychotics has been to develop medications that are more effective and safer, and this has happened rapidly, however, with underwhelming results. After the introduction of clozapine to the U.S. market around 1990, over the next decade at least three atypical antipsychotics were developed, approved, and marketed in the United States: risperidone, olanzapine, and quetiapine. When they first came out, there was great hope that they would change the way that psychosis was treated and transform patients' lives.

It was originally thought that olanzapine, which utilizes the same basic chemical structure that clozapine does, would be as effective in treating treatment-resistant psychosis. Unfortunately, it was quickly found that olanzapine's effectiveness was similar to risperidone and quetiapine, which were all less effective than clozapine. As medications were marketed and found to be less effective than hoped, the push and drive continued to develop atypicals that would behave more like clozapine, without the risk of agranulocytosis.

Between 2001 and 2010, there were at least six second-generation antipsychotics that were approved by the Food and Drug Administration (FDA) and put out on the market. While some of those newer antipsychotics have been found to be effective in a certain patient population, none of them have been found to behave as clozapine does; none are as effective for use in treatment-resistant psychosis; they have not been found to be as beneficial as hoped in treating negative symptoms; and while they may have less affinity to cause movement side effects, they all have been found to have a burdensome metabolic side effect profile.

The biggest shift in treatment of psychosis came in the early 1950s, with the introduction of the first antipsychotic, chlorpromazine. That was an exciting time for the treatment of psychotic disorders, and it changed the way mental illness was viewed and addressed. Over the decades that followed it became clear that still people with schizophrenia continued to be overrepresented among the non-married, childless, unemployed, underemployed, and low academic achievers. The cost of schizophrenia in both human and financial terms is great to society, individuals, and families, and while the introduction of antipsychotics greatly impacted positive symptoms, they failed in all of these other areas of treatment. Throughout the past decades, numerous antipsychotics have been developed in attempts to better treatment; however, when looking at them as a whole, there has been relatively little advancement in the field. Discovery platforms have repeatedly produced drugs with the same or similar mechanisms of action. After more than 60 years of drug development, only one medication has been shown to have superior efficacy in treating psychosis, and no medications have been found to really address any of the symptoms of chronic psychotic disorders other than the positive psychotic symptoms. All of this leads to a continued inadequacy in addressing quality of life and functional outcomes with antipsychotic medications.

One of the reasons the development of antipsychotics has traveled this path is likely because the positive symptoms of psychosis became the defining feature of chronic psychotic disorders. For that reason, clinical trials for antipsychotics used primary endpoints that would reflect improvements in positive psychotic symptoms as therapeutically effective. This inherently led to further development of antipsychotics that targeted and were effective in treating positive psychotic symptoms. At some point there was a slow, and now continuing, shift in how the disorder was conceptualized. It changed from a single disease view to a multi-domain pathological disorder and became more important to understand the various domains of the disorder, as they may respond to different types of treatment. There are three domains considered that can then be broken down even further: positive psychotic symptoms, negative symptoms, and pathology in interpersonal relating. These three domains have been broken down and specified even further in ways that will hopefully be beneficial for drug development. As they become more specific, it is more feasible to develop animal and human experimental models to address the domains, including impaired cognition and negative symptoms. Part of the issue remains that chronic psychotic disorders are complex, multidimensional disorders that are not well understood at the molecular level, making it difficult to develop medications to target the various domains of the disorder.

PATHOPHYSIOLOGY OF CHRONIC PSYCHOTIC DISORDERS

The industry has failed to identify key molecular pathologic elements as treatment targets. Meaning, basic knowledge of the molecular etiology of the disorder and of the symptoms is not adequate, which makes it very difficult to develop drugs that have a high predictive validity for success. The information known thus far about chronic psychotic disorders is really based on the idea that positive psychotic symptoms are the identifying feature of the disease, as opposed to looking at the other domains of the disorder and understanding the pathophysiology in each area of the disorder. For many diseases, the development of medications to treat them comes first from an understanding of how the disease attacks the body at a molecular level. There is a need to understand first, normal physiology and then to understand what happens in a pathological situation, pathophysiology. If there is a clear understanding of the disease process at a molecular level in the body, then a medication can be developed with confidence that it can interact at that molecular level and be therapeutic. This level of understanding is not present for many of the psychiatric illnesses, including chronic psychotic disorder, partly because the disease process in many disorders seems to be more complex than just a molecular change or impairment, as mentioned earlier when discussing the various domains of schizophrenia. However, this has been and will continue to be an area of interest for the development of new antipsychotics. The difference now and moving forward seems to be that the focus is not just on understanding the pathophysiology of positive psychotic symptoms, but trying to gain greater understanding of the pathophysiology at a molecular level for both the negative symptoms and cognitive impairments associated with the disorder. If this can be understood better, then medications can be developed that target these areas of deficit more specifically and have a higher probability of being effective therapeutically in those domains.

Genetics

For many psychiatric illnesses, the heritability is unclear; however, for both bipolar disorder and schizophrenia, there is clearly some genetic heritability. A current area of interest in drug development revolves around this idea, utilizing genetic studies in order to develop novel drug treatments. This area of study was greatly advanced in 2003 when the Human Genome Project was completed. A genome is an organism's complete set of DNA. The Human Genome Project was an international research effort to determine the sequence of the human genome and identify all of the genes that it contains. It is basically the blueprint to create a functional human being. The project was completed in 2003 and has many implications for the medical field. While for most diseases heredity is only one of the factors that contributes to a person's overall risk of developing the disease or disorder, genomics can be helpful in identifying those at risk of the disorder and help with preventative measures. More importantly, for the purposes of this book, genomics is an ever-growing field that is thought to be greatly beneficial in the development of new medications. With genomics, there will be the ability to not only identify patients who may be at risk of developing a disorder, but clinical researchers may also be able to develop drugs to target specific gene variants. The field is also likely to help allow the prediction of an individual's responsiveness to a certain medication, even within the same class as another medication, as variations in responsiveness are thought due to genetic differences. For example, it may be found that there are a number of different gene variants (variation from the normal gene) that are associated with schizophrenia. And it then could be found that risperidone is very effective in targeting gene variant 1 and aripiprazole is effective in targeting gene variant 2. This information can then be utilized to individualize a person's treatment and to get higher levels of responsiveness to medications. This is one way that genomics could help to push treatment with antipsychotics into the future, into a more individualized and effective treatment. However, it will also hopefully assist in the development of novel antipsychotics or other medications to address the cognitive deficits and negative psychotic symptoms. The hope is that by using genomics, researchers can gain a greater understanding of the genetic variants that can lead to development of the disorder or at least increase risk of development of the disorder. With that understanding, novel drug therapies that target the specific genetic variant could be developed.

The previous pages discuss some of the main areas where antipsychotics are currently failing and where some of the research may be heading. It is clear, and has been clear for some years now, that the biggest areas of failure in treatment revolve around negative psychotic symptoms and cognitive impairments. That has not changed. Part of that failure is paralleled in the development of antipsychotics that all have very similar mechanisms of action. The potential of genomics use in individualizing treatment and developing novel treatments is real but still in the early stages of development. So what else is going on currently to advance the treatment of psychosis? What medications are currently being studied, and do they offer any divergence from the current antipsychotics that we have? These are some of the questions that will be addressed in the following pages to get a further understanding of what the future of this class of medications is shaping up to be.

NEW MEDICATIONS ON THE HORIZON

At any given time, there are multiple medications under various stages of development, attempting to be the next "breakthrough" medication for psychosis. Instead of discussing specific medications that may currently be in different stages of trials, it would be more beneficial to understand what types of medications are being looked at for development. There are still, of course, medications being researched as antipsychotics that block dopamine as their main mechanism of action. If the past predicts the future, then likely, these medications will not prove to be more therapeutically efficacious and will probably have their own set of burdensome side effects. But still it is easier to try to make smaller changes to a mechanism of action that has already proven to be somewhat successful than to "recreate the wheel." Some of these medications may provide alternatives or be more tolerable than the antipsychotics that already exist. However, more interestingly, there are medications being researched that have entirely different mechanisms of action than blocking dopamine, which would be new to the field of antipsychotics. Some of the more promising hypotheses involve the role of acetylcholine, glutamate, gamma-aminobutyric acid (GABA), and serotonin in schizophrenia, which will be discussed in the following pages.

Acetylcholine Agonists

Acetylcholine is a neurotransmitter that is found both in the central nervous system (brain and spinal cord) and the peripheral nervous system (nerves outside the brain and spinal cord) and that plays a role in a variety of functions, including, but not limited to, sensory, motor, attention, mood, and cognitive processing. There are two different types of acetylcholine receptors, muscarinic and nicotinic, that differ in function and structure, and in the past decade, there has been some attention paid to muscarinic acetylcholine receptors and their potential role in schizophrenia. This hypothesis has been based on data found from postmortem studies, neuroimaging, and clinical and preclinical pharmacology studies. Postmortem and neuroimaging studies have shown a decrease in two types of muscarinic acetylcholine receptors in people with schizophrenia that is not seen in people with other psychiatric illnesses.

Medications that increase acetylcholine are often used to treat Alzheimer's disease, and they are used to improve cognitive functioning, which suggests that acetylcholine agonists may lead to cognitive improvements. Medications that block muscarinic receptors have been found to cause cognitive dysfunction in healthy individuals as well as people with schizophrenia and have been associated with a worsening of positive psychotic symptoms and improvement in negative psychotic symptoms. These data do not clearly show the impact of muscarinic acetylcholine receptors on schizophrenia, but these do seem to show that muscarinic activity is associated with changes in psychotic symptoms and cognitive symptoms, giving good reason for further research into its potential role in pathology and treatment. There has been some evidence that synthetic muscarinic acetylcholine receptor agonists (in particular agonists of the type of receptor found to be decreased in schizophrenia) lead to an improvement in positive symptoms as well as cognitive function. Some medications already developed and approved for treatment in Alzheimer's disease are now being studied for treatment of schizophrenia. Also, because of this hypothesis and data connecting acetylcholine and psychosis, there are new medications currently under development meant to act at the muscarinic acetylcholine receptors, leading to an increase in acetylcholine that may lead to new antipsychotic medications. However, acetylcholine is not the only neurotransmitter hypothesized to be involved in psychosis and schizophrenia. For the field of antipsychotic treatment, this is probably a good thing. It does mean that still, there is an unclear understanding of how schizophrenia is operating, but it means that there are multiple mechanisms being explored, which makes it more likely there will be development of a medication approved to treat psychosis that does not impact dopamine.

Glutamate and Psychosis

The hypothesis that glutamate is involved in the development of schizophrenia was proposed around two decades ago; however, it has continued to develop and has expanded over the years. And still the main mechanism of action for all antipsychotics involves dopamine, suggesting that there is more research to be done with other neurotransmitters. Glutamate is another neurotransmitter, abundant in the brain. It is involved in many aspects of normal brain function, including cognition, memory, and learning. It is considered the major mediator of excitatory signals in the brain. The hypothesis for glutamate's role in schizophrenia came after it was observed that drugs that blocked certain glutamate receptors were found to induce psychosis and schizophrenia-like symptoms. It has since been expanded to suggest that abnormalities in the glutamate system may disturb normal functions and lead to psychosis and cognitive disturbances. There have been studies attempting to link changes in glutamate with psychosis that have shown associations between glutamate levels and various psychotic symptoms. It is suggested that glutamate levels may be selectively elevated in those whose positive symptoms are not well controlled by current antipsychotic treatment. This is not clearly suggesting that glutamate is the only neurotransmitter involved and suggests perhaps a more complicated picture with interactions of multiple neurotransmitters.

Similarly, there is some conflicting evidence when looking at glutamate and negative symptoms, with some studies showing higher levels of glutamate with more severe negative symptoms, some showing lower levels of glutamate, and some showing no significant relationship at all. The other domain to consider when looking at a neurotransmitter's potential impact on schizophrenia is the cognitive domain. In this domain as well there is inconsistent evidence thus far as to the specific role and impact of glutamate with cognitive functioning; however, it does seem that there is some role and further research to clarify that would be beneficial. Studies have also looked at an area of schizophrenia that is not always considered when thinking about hypothesis of pathology, social and occupational functioning. Several studies have shown that in first-episode psychosis and chronic schizophrenia, higher glutamate levels in particular areas of the brain have been associated with worse overall social and occupational functioning.

The data that have been found about glutamate and schizophrenia do not point to a clear hypothesis of its involvement in the disorder; however the data do show many associations to the disorder and suggest some type of role in the symptoms. Because of this there is a need for further research into its role, and already there are medications that act on glutamate receptors that are under development for treatment of psychosis. Likely because the role is not as defined, there are also many medications under development that do not act directly on glutamate receptors but have some effect on glutamate levels in the brain.

GABA

GABA is another neurotransmitter found throughout the central nervous system. It can be thought of as the counterpart to glutamate as it is considered the major inhibitory neurotransmitter and has also been hypothesized to play a role in the development of schizophrenia. This hypothesis for GABA's role in schizophrenia goes back all the way to the 1970s, when it was hypothesized that GABA had a role interacting with dopamine in the development of schizophrenia. The hypothesis has gone in and out of favor in the field and has developed and been modified throughout the years. More recently, it has been suggested that deficits in GABA are linked to symptoms of cognitive dysfunction in schizophrenia, and there are studies that show that people with schizophrenia have reduced GABA concentration in certain brain areas. There are studies showing that induction of a GABA-deficient state leads to vulnerability in healthy individuals for induction of psychosis if using drugs that are known to cause it. One of the differences between the GABA hypothesis and others is that there is a consistent suggestion that the role of GABA might be an interaction with dopamine. It seems more that the data show that GABA might help protect against development of schizophrenia or psychosis, and if there is a deficit, then one is just more vulnerable to developing a disorder that may be caused or impacted by a different neurotransmitter. There are studies that show abnormalities in GABA in people with schizophrenia, suggesting that GABA agonists could be beneficial, but generally the implication is not that a GABA agonist would be the main treatment, but that it would be considered adjunctive and could be added on to a current antipsychotic that works on dopamine.

Serotonin

Serotonin is another neurotransmitter found not only throughout the central nervous system but also in the gut and on blood cells. It has many functions but is primarily thought of as having a role in regulating mood. As mentioned earlier in the book, it is thought to have a role in psychotic symptoms. Its role in schizophrenia has been hypothesized for some time now, and while the main hypothesis continues to be dopamine, there seems to be a consensus that it is more complex than that and that serotonin plays a role somehow. To speak to that, there are many antipsychotics that have some activity at serotonin receptors; however, there are not antipsychotics that have a primary mechanism of action involving serotonin. There are, though, multiple medications currently under development that are looking at the potential for a serotonin antagonist as the primary mechanism of action for an antipsychotic. Some of the most convincing evidence that serotonin does play a role in schizophrenia comes from the effectiveness of some of the atypical antipsychotics like clozapine and risperidone. Both of those medications may be better serotonin antagonists than dopamine antagonists and are effective at treating schizophrenia, suggesting strongly that serotonin at the very least plays a role in the disorder.

Acetylcholine, glutamate, GABA, and serotonin are all neurotransmitters that have been hypothesized to have some impact on psychosis for some time now. Further research on their involvement and on new medication development is currently in process and offers some hope for a new line of antipsychotics. There are other compounds that have more recently been suggested to be associated with psychosis, including histamine and oxytocin, both of which also are being researched as potential novel treatments.

Histamine

Histamine is a compound that is not only well known for its involvement in local immune responses, but it also works in the gut and as a neurotransmitter. As a neurotransmitter, histamine plays a role in the sleep-wake cycle by increasing wakefulness and preventing sleep, which is why sometimes antihistamines are used to help with sleep difficulties. However, it is also thought to play a role as a neurotransmitter in schizophrenia as its metabolites have been found to be increased in the cerebrospinal fluid of people with schizophrenia. Because of this, some of the more recent antipsychotics have antihistaminic properties as secondary mechanisms of action, but there are no medications currently approved that use histamine antagonism as the primary mechanism of action. Over the past decade, the functional role of histamine as a neurotransmitter has become more clarified, including its major role in control of arousal, cognition, and energy balance. There are a number of studies that have shown an association between increased histamine and psychosis. Some animal studies have shown an increase in histamine activity in the brain after administration of some of the psychosis-inducing drugs like methamphetamine or N-methyl-D-aspartate (NMDA) antagonists. Other animal models have shown antipsychotic properties with histamine blockers, but there is limited predictive value in animal studies when trying to determine how efficacious they will be in human models. Therefore, more research is needed with antihistamines as antipsychotics in humans, which is underway. There are more medications being developed that utilize antihistaminic properties as secondary mechanisms of action, and there are some being developed that are attempting to utilize them as the primary mechanism of action, which could prove to be a novel antipsychotic treatment.

Oxytocin

Another compound that has more recently gained interest for its potential role in psychosis and as a potential form of treatment is oxytocin. Oxytocin is a hormone, neuropeptide, and medication. As a neuropeptide, it is a molecule used to communicate among neurons. Oxytocin has a very wide variety of functions ranging from uterine contraction, to breastfeeding, to prosocial behaviors, which is where it may be linked to the development and treatment of schizophrenia. It plays a role in modulating social behavior, increasing trust, and decreasing social distance between males and females and is thought to assist in facilitating trust and attachment between individuals. Oxytocin has been studied in animals and shown to have prosocial and antipsychotic-like effects. It has started to be studied in humans and thus far has shown some promising effect. Its primary route of administration is intranasally, which is new, and some evidence supports it causing a decrease in positive psychotic symptoms, a decrease in negative psychotic symptoms, and improvement in several social cognition measures. This is a potentially novel new treatment that could provide new effectiveness in the negative symptoms and cognitive symptoms that has not been seen before. Currently there is a drug company that has branded intranasal oxytocin, and its research is in phase II clinical trials. This means it has already been a part of a small research group to determine safety, side effects, and dosage range. It is now being tested on a larger group of people to determine its effectiveness and further evaluate safety. While oxytocin has the potential to add exciting new treatment benefits, it is not currently being studied as a primary mode of treatment but would be used as an add-on medication to address some of the symptoms that are not managed well by current antipsychotics.

Currently one of the major areas where antipsychotics are coming up short is in the treatment of chronic psychotic disorders as a multi-domain illness. Notably they are failing to appropriately address both cognitive impairment and negative symptoms. This has been on the minds of people in the field for decades, and currently, as mentioned earlier, there are multiple novel medications under research that hope to address these two functional limiting domains. Another question one could ask is how to make improvements in the antipsychotics that are already available? While the typical and atypical antipsychotics are relatively effective in treating positive psychotic symptoms, there is still a fairly high rate of noncompliance, which leads to decompensation of psychotic symptoms. One of the current and future directions of movement for antipsychotics is exploring other routes of administration, which will be discussed next.

BETTER ROUTES OF ADMINISTRATION

After antipsychotics were discovered in the 1950s, poor adherence to the oral medication was found to be a critical issue, so other routes were considered. The first long-acting injectable was developed in 1966, fluphenazine enanthate, and haloperidol decanoate became available in the United States in 1986. Clinical results were great, and a large reduction in the morbidity of chronic psychotic disorders was seen. However, initially, this route of treatment was not well received by the public or the medical field, partly because of concern of side effects and partly because of fear that it was imposing treatment on people who may not want it. Soon after their introduction, however, their clinical use proved to be quite beneficial, and they became quite popular. As antipsychotics have continued in their development, long-acting injectables have been developed for multiple atypical antipsychotics along with the typical antipsychotics, and many patients find them to be a more desirable alternative to taking a pill every day.

Just think about how difficult it is to remember to take a pill every day, for example, a vitamin. The goal is taking one each day, but occasionally you might miss one, and then one becomes a few and then it is difficult to get back into that routine. Now imagine that you have been diagnosed with an illness that impacts your sense of reality, motivation, and cognitive functioning. You are supposed to take a pill every day, which is hard enough to remember, but then you miss it one day and you do not notice much of a difference, so you keep taking it some days, but it becomes not as important because it does not seem to change when you do not take it. So then you decide to just stop taking it because it does not seem to matter if you miss one here or there, or it just becomes less important and you stop taking it a for a number of days in a row. Now next thing you know your family is acting concerned about you, you begin to isolate yourself and start hearing a voice telling you not to take your medication and then you end up in the hospital. For people with chronic psychotic illnesses, it can be very difficult to take a pill every day for years and years. When someone misses their daily vitamin here and there, the consequences are minimal to absent, but when someone misses their antipsychotic, the consequences can be severe, leading to dangerous acts, hospitalization, and/or worsening of the illness. The long-acting injectables have changed that and made lives much easier for a number of people suffering with mental illnesses, but there might still be room for improvement.

Current Long-Acting Injectables

Currently there are at least six forms of antipsychotics that are available in a long-acting injectable form. Some of these are easier to utilize in clinical care than others, and some last for two weeks, while others last for four weeks. There are two typical antipsychotic forms of long-acting injectables, one of which is haloperidol decanoate, which is probably used more often than the fluphenazine decanoate. Both are relatively cheap and neither of them requires that they be stored in refrigeration, like some of the others do, but fluphenazine is dosed every two to four weeks and haloperidol is dosed every four weeks. Likely because of the extended length of the dosing, haloperidol decanoate is used more frequently. Then there are at least four atypical antipsychotics that have developed long-acting injectable forms of delivery. They include risperidone, olanzapine, paliperidone, and aripiprazole. While risperidone is a commonly used oral medication, it is more difficult to use in the long-acting injectable form than some of the others. Risperidone's long-acting injectable form requires that it be stored in a refrigerated area, which is sometimes difficult to do as the patient has to go to a clinic to get the injection. So the medication either has to be stored refrigerated at a clinic or the patient would have to be responsible for picking up the medication and storing it refrigerated at home and bringing it to the clinic appointment. Also this form has to be given every two weeks, which makes it slightly less desirable. Out of all of the long-acting injectables available, currently the longest working medications need to be given every four weeks. When you compare that with taking a medication every day, or even getting an injection every two weeks, that sounds like a good option. But when you consider that we are capable of making a medication available in the body for four weeks, one may ask, why not longer? Can we make a long-acting injectable that only has to be given every two months? Or maybe every six months or even every year? And once you start asking those questions, you also have to consider what is an ethically and medically appropriate length of time for a medication to be available in the body after a one-time dose.

Long-Acting Injectables in the Future

As mentioned previously, it took some time for the long-acting injectables to be accepted in the medical field as well as with the lay public. While they are currently more accepted and utilized, there is certainly room to grow. There are a number of studies that demonstrate the economic and personal cost that comes from a chronic course of a psychotic illness that often includes many episodes of decompensation, usually associated with stopping a medication. Once a medication is stopped and a person decompensates, he or she often requires hospitalization, which costs the person and society both money and emotional hardships. Using long-acting injectables has been shown to decrease emergency department visits as well as decrease in the number of rehospitalizations in patients with an established diagnosis of schizophrenia. Therefore, one future direction for antipsychotics is simply the continued and increased use and development of more long-acting injectables. These have already shown to impact positively the emotional and financial cost of schizophrenia, so making them more readily available and less stigmatized is an easy step to help progress the treatment of chronic psychosis. Currently general practice is to consider the use of long-term injectables after a course of schizophrenia has already been established. Still, they are not generally discussed in treatment unless a patient expresses an interest in something other than a daily oral medication or the patient has had multiple episodes of stopping the oral medication, which led to adverse events and/or return of distressing symptoms. Even the most recent American Psychiatric Association's (APA) practice guidelines for the treatment of schizophrenia suggest that most patients prefer oral medication but that those who prefer injectables should be offered them as well as patients with recurrent relapses related to medication nonadherence. The wording of the guidelines seems to almost discourage providers from discussing the options of long-acting injectables with many of their patients who are suffering from a chronic psychotic illness. However, there seems to be some type of attitude shift in the field toward long-acting injectables, which is slowly developing. Many clinicians are expressing more and more interest in the use and benefit of this route of administration, especially as more forms of the injectables, specifically atypical antipsychotics, become available.

Still, most of the research has been done with a population that has a clearly defined chronic relapsing course of the psychotic illness. And in this population, the use of the long-term injectables has been shown to provide great benefit in the clinical course. Currently, this route of medication is usually considered once a lot of damage has already been done, which leads to the question: should it be considered earlier on in the course of the disease in order to prevent nonadherence which leads to relapse and greater cost to the patient?

In the past 5–10 years, there has been a much greater awareness and amount of attention, both in the mental health field and in the public, paid to the "first break." This is a term used to describe the first psychotic episode, which often occurs in late adolescence and can lead to a chronic course of a debilitating psychotic disorder. Generally an adolescent will experience a first psychotic episode of schizophrenia around the time he or she should be graduating high school, working a first job, or attending college. This can be detrimental to the patient's functioning, and it is often, understandably, difficult to accept by both the patient and family members. This can lead to some type of denial that can then lead to medication and treatment nonadherence, which only furthers the impact of the disorder on the patient's functioning and can be the beginning of a heartbreaking disorder and life course for the individual and family and friends. The shift in the field has been toward really targeting that time in a patient's life and treatment in order to help preserve functioning and treat early in order to support both the patient and the family to help change the course of the illness and its impact. As this becomes a priority in the mental health field, there is a growing interest in the potential for long-acting injectables to be used in this patient population. There have been some studies looking at the use of long-acting injectables in this population, generally looking at the atypical antipsychotics, and thus far, they have shown promising results. Studies have tried to look at the use of the long-acting injectables in patients with recent-onset schizophrenia to see if their implementation would show a benefit not only in clinical symptoms but also in social and occupational functioning, quality of life, and hospital readmission rates. Many of the studies seem to show some improvement in all of these areas; however, most of the studies have many limitations with small sample sizes or the lack of a compared group, and many are not randomized controlled trials. Thus the suggestion is that in the future, this long-acting injectable form of antipsychotics may be more applicable to a wider patient population than it is currently being targeted to, and it has the potential to positively impact the current huge burden that this disease carries for both individuals and society.

The idea that long-acting injectable antipsychotics could reach a larger population and provide benefit makes one question what other changes could be made to routes of administration that may benefit those suffering from psychosis. Long-acting injectables could be extended to become longer-release formulations, but there are other modes of delivery that may be just as beneficial or more beneficial. Think about how other medications can be delivered to a person when he or she needs to be taking them in the long term. People with allergies spray their medication in their nose every day. Is this a possibility for antipsychotics? And would it bring any novel and beneficial attributes to the treatment? People with nicotine addiction, chronic pain, and dementia can use patches that are placed on the arm or back to deliver their medication through their skin. Is it possible that there is role for this in antipsychotic delivery? Some people who need vascular stents or stimulators to certain parts of the body like the heart or the spine get implants in their body to help deliver treatment. People with diabetes can get an insulin pump implanted that delivers the insulin needed to the body. Is this a potential option for route of delivery of antipsychotics? All of these methods of delivery are meant to assist with those who have chronic need for medical treatment in an attempt to improve adherence and make treatment easier. While all of these are potential areas of research for developing new routes of administration for antipsychotics, the most relevant currently is the intranasal route.

Intranasal Antipsychotics

Earlier in this chapter, it was briefly mentioned that oxytocin is a new drug under development for treatment of schizophrenia that can be delivered intranasally. This means, just like the allergy medicine that others spray in each nostril every day, that one would spray the medication in their nostril as opposed to taking a pill each day. This route of administration is one that has been gaining more popularity in research in mental health over the past decade. Why, one might ask, would it be more beneficial to spray your medicine up your nostril every day instead of taking a pill? Is it easier? For those who have difficulty swallowing a pill, it might be easier or for those who do not like the taste that some medications can leave in their mouth. But those folks are likely in the minority. And as discussed earlier, one of the biggest issues with oral medication is having to remember to take it every day, so the intranasal route of administration offers no benefit or advantage in that domain. There is still a stigma attached to mental illness, especially with psychotic disorders; so does taking your medication through your nostril as opposed to a pill every day decrease or remove some of that stigma? That seems possible but still unclear.

The main reason that intranasal route of administration is intriguing to those developing and marketing medications is because it is believed that intranasal route offers both direct and indirect pathways to deliver the medications to the central nervous system. It suggests that if medication is given through the nostril, it will make it to the brain, the primary end point, faster and perhaps with greater effect than if it has to travel there after being absorbed through the gastrointestinal (GI) system. Getting medication to the brain is always challenging, especially for certain types of medications, because the brain is somewhat delicate and essential and so it is protected. The brain has a barrier called the blood-brain barrier that is a permeable barrier (meaning it allows some things to pass through it, but it is highly selective in what is able to pass). The barrier separates the circulating blood from the extracellular fluid that flows through the central nervous system. The barrier is meant to protect the brain from damaging molecules that may try to pass through. There is a reason that some drugs of abuse are snorted, and medications are no exception. Like drugs of abuse, medications that are given in the nose are absorbed through the nasal epithelium and are immediately absorbed into the systemic blood circulation. This leads to them making it to the brain and causing effect quite quickly, as opposed to other medications that are taken orally and then must travel through the GI system and be absorbed through the GI system and work their way up to the blood-brain barrier. If antipsychotics could be developed that could be used intranasally, perhaps they could be more targeted, would work faster, and would decrease the GI side effects that are seen with some of them.

One of the other ways that intranasal antipsychotics could prove to be beneficial would be in emergent situations. Currently there are few options when a person is in a psychotic state and becomes agitated and dangerous to himself or herself or others around. Oral antipsychotics will work eventually, but they do not give relief immediately, so more is generally needed in an emergency. Historically, if people were acutely psychotic and agitated and were putting themselves or others at risk, they would be physically restrained. Those physical restraints included tying people down to their beds in order to help prevent harm. Thankfully, as societal views have changed and more options for treatment have become available, this is not a widely used practice anymore, and many states have regulations about how any kind of restraint can be used and their use is monitored. Patients can receive short-acting injections of antipsychotics in an emergent situation if there is concern for risk to the patient or others, which is, to say the least, not the most desirable scenario. The injectable form of the antipsychotic works much faster than the oral form and may provide some relief to the patient and help to keep others safe, but it is an invasion of a person's body and has its own risks that come with a forced injection. If there were an option to give an intranasal form of an antipsychotic in an emergent situation with an acutely psychotic patient, that could be much more desirable for all involved, still producing fast results and minimizing risk and harm to all involved.

Thus far, we have discussed where antipsychotics are falling short, some of the new and novel medications that are under development, new ways to use already existing antipsychotics, and new routes of administration, all of which are on the horizon for antipsychotics and treatment; however, this has focused mainly on the treatment of chronic psychotic disorders. The future of antipsychotics in the use of nonpsychotic disorders is growing and gaining momentum quickly.

USE IN NONPSYCHOTIC DISORDERS

Initially, antipsychotics were used almost solely for primary psychotic disorders; their efficacy in some other disorders has slowly been identified, but over the past two decades, their use in many other disorders has grown drastically and will likely continue to flourish. Bipolar disorder can have a psychotic component, yet it does not have to. Antipsychotics have been approved for some realm of treatment in bipolar disorder for a number of years, and with continued and greater use, it has been found that many of the antipsychotic agents are maybe even more beneficial in the depressed phase of bipolar disorder than the traditional treatments, the mood stabilizers. This would lead to a curiosity about antipsychotics and their potential use in unipolar depression. For some time now there has been good evidence that combining an antipsychotic with an antidepressant for the treatment of psychotic depression is more beneficial than either class of medication used on its own. But for many years it was not so clear that perhaps antipsychotics could serve as augmenters to nonpsychotic unipolar depression, meaning depression without manic symptoms or psychotic symptoms. Starting in the mid-2000s, second-generation antipsychotics began getting FDA approval for adjunctive treatment of unipolar depression. Aripiprazole was the first in 2007, meaning that if a patient were suffering from depression and not responding to antidepressants, it would be FDA-approved to add aripiprazole to the antidepressant to target the depressive symptoms. After aripiprazole, more atypical antipsychotics sought approval and gained it and have shown clear data that they are effective and maybe more effective than other medications that have been used in the past as adjunctive treatments. One of the atypical antipsychotics, Seroquel XR (extended release formulation), has even been approved to treat depression on its own, without adding an antidepressant. According to the National Institute of Mental Health (NIMH), in the United States, in 2014, the prevalence of major depression was 6.7%, meaning that approximately 15.7 million adults had at least one major depressive episode that year. This disorder has a high cost to society as a whole and is lacking in good treatment, specifically for those who do not respond to first-line antidepressants, which is why the potential for antipsychotics to be beneficial to that group is exciting. Further studies with already existing antipsychotics and their role in depression as well as development of new antipsychotics that may target depression more directly are on the horizon.

Anxiety disorders are another area where more recently antipsychotics have been considered in augmenting their treatment. Quetiapine has been studied the most, specifically in controlled trials for the treatment of generalized anxiety disorder. Trials have shown that quetiapine is effective in treating generalized anxiety disorder and is comparable in efficacy to other medications that have FDA approval for the treatment of generalized anxiety. However, the FDA recommended against approval of quetiapine at this time because of safety concerns, meaning that the risks of the side effects, mostly the metabolic side effects, of quetiapine were considered to be too high or dangerous compared to the benefit that people would receive by taking the medication, especially since there are already FDA-approved medications with less risky side effect profiles and similar efficacy. One potential advantage of antipsychotics in the treatment of anxiety disorders is their more rapid onset of action. Recall that antipsychotics generally begin taking effect within the first week of treatment. However, most antidepressants, which are first-line treatment for anxiety disorders, generally take 4–12 weeks to show effect. While quetiapine was not FDA-approved, this is promising for the future of antipsychotic use in anxiety disorders and will need to be studied further and will likely be considered in the development of new antipsychotics.

As noted earlier in the book, antipsychotics are currently used for a number of other disorders, including, but not limited to, agitation in the elderly, impulsive disorders of childhood, and autism. Some antipsychotics have very limited FDA approval in some of these disorders like autism spectrum disorder; however, as time goes on and more studies and trials are conducted, there will be a drive to find uses for antipsychotics in other disorders, especially disorders with impulsivity as a major component. One of the areas that antipsychotics are currently used, but there is lacking research, is in the domain of personality disorders. Some of the personality disorders have a schizophrenic feel without the positive psychotic symptoms, and antipsychotics can be used to help improve functioning in that patient population. There is also a group of personality disorders that include a great deal of mood dysregulation, aggression, and impulsivity. Atypical antipsychotics are used frequently with this population, and there is an improvement in aggression and impulsivity that is seen, but studies are lacking. Moving forward, more research will be done in these areas to help find approved treatment for some of these disorders. In general, as the atypical antipsychotics have continued to develop, because they have multiple mechanisms of action, they have been found to be effective in targeting a variety of symptoms. In the past one to two decades, this has become clearer as they have begun getting approval for other disorders like autism and depression. This is likely just the beginning for their development, and further research will include medications that still not only have true antipsychotic properties but also target other symptoms like anxiety, impulsivity, irritability, and social withdrawal and will therefore be able to expand and broaden their use.

Broadening the use of antipsychotics is the future of antipsychotics. This book started at the beginning of antipsychotics, or even before, determining a need for antipsychotics. It traveled through the history and development of some of the individual drugs and the class of medications as a whole. Their use was strictly defined as a medication to treat the positive symptoms of psychosis for many years. And when they were originally developed, that was a much needed treatment. They served that purpose, and will continue to do so, but as society and the mental health field have developed as well, the need has changed. The development of antipsychotics was groundbreaking for mental health treatment at the time, but then they basically stood still for many years, with only clozapine standing out as any real advancement for decades. Similarly mental health, specifically psychotic disorders, and its standing in society has developed and changed—first viewed as a problem that should be locked away and removed from society, changing to an issue that should be living amongst society and treated in the community whenever at all possible. Our developments in antipsychotics have lagged behind our ideas and ideals about how it should be treated. Currently, antipsychotics are reasonably good at treating positive psychotic symptoms but fail to address any of the other psychotic symptoms or impacts. But over the past one to two decades, there has been growing awareness for the need of development of more novel antipsychotic treatments and augmenters for antipsychotics in schizophrenia. Both of these are promising in suggesting there will be more push and research into the development of more novel treatments. There is also more attention being paid to the younger generation, onset of chronic psychotic disorders in adolescence, and the need to be treating early and considering alternative medications and routes of administration.

One of the battles that antipsychotics have faced and continue to face, along with the rest of mental health, is that of the stigma associated with mental illnesses. This too has been an ongoing and ever-developing and changing aspect related to mental health treatment. There is continued push and efforts to help destigmatize mental illness and its treatment and that has been somewhat successful over the years, but the stigma still exists. This has influenced why there was little to no movement in the development of antipsychotics for so many years. As the stigma decreases, society and individuals become more open to antipsychotics as treatment, which means there is more money to put into research to develop more novel treatments. By no means has stigma gone away and likely never will completely, but it has decreased over the years, which is encouraging for the future of antipsychotics and the future of those suffering with mental illnesses.

The future of antipsychotics is bright and rich. The class of medications was somewhat stagnant for a number of years, and over the past 15 years, there has been life renewed into their development. In the coming years, it is likely we will see multiple more atypical antipsychotics, similar to the ones already on the market, approved by the FDA. Along with that there will likely be some that have different mechanisms of action and are even composed of highly different compounds than what is currently on the market. They will probably be approved to treat a much wider range of disorders, including depression and aggression. We will see antipsychotics that can be delivered via new routes of administration, which in turn allow for more flexibility and opportunity to be making shared care decisions between the doctor and the patient. With more advances in antipsychotics, there is only more room for conversations to be taking place between doctors and patients about patient preferences, more space for patients to have more of a voice in their treatment. Finally, as this seems to be the main focus and hole in current antipsychotic treatment, there will be some new development in a current medication or new medications that will target the negative psychotic symptoms and cognitive impairments from chronic psychotic disorders that are so debilitating for both the individual and society as a whole.

Directory of Resources

CENTERS FOR MEDICARE AND MEDICAID SERVICES (CMS)

7500 Security Boulevard
Baltimore, MD 21244
www.cms.gov

CMS is part of the Department of Health and Human Services that administers programs such as Medicare, Medicaid, the Children's Health Insurance Program, and the Health Insurance Marketplace. They work to strengthen and modernize the U.S. health-care system while providing quality care at lower costs by utilizing value-based incentives, improving payment models, and tying payment to better outcomes.

CLOZAPINE REMS (RISK EVALUATION AND MITIGATION STRATEGIES)

Clozapine REMS Program
PO Box 2058
Phoenix, AZ 85038-9058
844-267-8678
www.clozapineremes.com

Clozapine REMS is a single shared program organizing the requirement to prescribe, dispense, and receive clozapine. The idea behind REMS is to ensure that the benefits of the drug outweigh the severe risks in each case, and this regulation is required by the Food and Drug Administration (FDA). The REMS program was initiated in 2015 and replaced the multiple individual clozapine patient registries that were formerly in use in the United States.

JUDGE DAVID L. BAZELON CENTER FOR MENTAL HEALTH LAW

The Bazelon Center for Mental Health Law
1101 15th Street, NW, Suite 1212
Washington, DC 20005
202-467-5730
communications@bazelon.org
www.bazelon.org

The Bazelon Center for Mental Health Law is a nonprofit organization that was founded in 1972 by a group of lawyers and professionals in mental health and mental disabilities whose mission is to protect and advance the rights of adults and children who have mental disabilities. Policy staffs promote goals of a progressive mental health policy agenda to reform systems and programs to protect the rights of children and adults with mental disabilities to lead lives with dignity in the community.

NATIONAL ALLIANCE ON MENTAL ILLNESS (NAMI)

3803 N. Fairfax Drive, Suite 100
Arlington, VA 22203
Main: 703-524-7600
Member Services: 888-999-6264
Helpline: 800-950-6264
www.nami.org

NAMI is the nation's largest grassroots mental health organization. It began as a small group of families in 1979 and now has hundreds of local affiliates, state organizations, and volunteers in communities working to raise awareness and provide support and education that have not been previously available. They offer educational programs throughout the country, advocate for people with mental illnesses and their families in public policy, offer a toll-free helpline, and have various public awareness events and activities.

NATIONAL INSTITUTE OF MENTAL HEALTH (NIMH)

Science Writing, Press, and Dissemination Branch
6001 Executive Boulevard, Room 6200, MSC 9663
Bethesda, MD 20892-9663
1-866-615-6464
nimhinfor@nih.gov
www.nimh.nih.gov

The NIMH is the lead federal agency for research on mental disorders. They envision a world in which mental illnesses are prevented and cured. The mission of NIMH is to transform the understanding and treatment of mental illnesses through basic and clinical research.

U.S. FOOD AND DRUG ADMINISTRATION

10903 New Hampshire Avenue
Silver Spring, MD 20993
1-888-INFO-FDA (1-888-463-6332)
www.fda.gov

The FDA is responsible for protecting the public health by ensuring that human and veterinary drugs and vaccines and other biological products and medical devices intended for human use are safe and effective. It is the major regulatory agency involved in the development, regulation, and marketing of both branded and generic prescription medications in the United States.

Glossary

Affect: The range and intensity of emotional response that a person expresses and that can be observed by another.

Agranulocytosis: A condition that leads to a dangerous lowering of the white blood cell count. More specifically it involves a decrease in neutrophils, which are one of the major types of white blood cells that fight infection in the body.

Akathisia: A movement disorder that is a side effect from a medication. It is characterized by an internal feeling of restlessness and a need to be in constant motion. People will often be pacing or simply moving from one foot to the other.

Anxiolytic: A medication used to decrease anxiety.

Arcuate nucleus: A group of neurons located in the hypothalamus that is part of the tuberoinfundibular pathway.

Autonomic nervous system: A system that is a division of the peripheral nervous system and works to unconsciously regulate bodily functions, including heart rate, digestion, sexual arousal, and respiratory rate, among others. It receives input from the limbic system and is primarily responsible for the fight-or-flight response.

Basal ganglia: Part of the brain made up of dorsal striatum, ventral striatum, globus pallidus, ventral pallidum, substantia nigra, and subthalamic nucleus. It is strongly connected to the cerebral cortex, thalamus, and brain stem. It houses many dopamine neurons and is strongly associated with the control of voluntary motor movements.

Benzodiazepine: A class of prescription medications used to treat anxiety, among other illnesses, that are sedating and also have abuse potential.

Black box warning: A warning put on prescription drugs or drug products by the FDA when there is evidence of an association of a serious hazard of the drug. It is the strictest warning used by the FDA and is designed to call attention to serious or life-threatening risks.

Body mass index: It is derived from someone's weight and height in an attempt to quantify the amount of tissue mass in an individual. After the calculation is done, a person can be categorized as underweight, normal, overweight, or obese. It is used in monitoring for metabolic syndrome and general health concerns associated with being underweight or overweight. Calculation: weight in pounds/height in inches squared × 703 or mass in kilograms/height in meters squared.

Central nervous system: The part of the nervous system that is made up of the brain and spinal cord.

Cerebral cortex: The outer layer of tissue on the brain, also known as gray matter. The cortex plays a role in memory, attention, perception, awareness, thought, language, and consciousness.

Circumstantiality: A non-linear thought pattern in which excessive details are often added. The thought strays from the original topic but eventually comes back around to the central theme.

Comorbidity: The presence of additional diseases co-occurring with a primary illness.

Delusion: A fixed, false belief that continues to be held with conviction despite contradictory evidence.

Dorsal striatum: A part of the forebrain that is critical to the reward system. It serves as the primary input to the basal ganglia and can be impacted in movement disorders.

Extrapyramidal symptoms: Drug-induced, often from antipsychotics, movement disorders. Caused by the drugs' actions in the extrapyramidal system, which regulates skeletal muscle tone and voluntary and involuntary movement.

Flight of ideas: A nonlinear thought process in which the responses are superficially associated, but the ideas rapidly shift from subject to subject. To the other participant in the conversation, it often sounds like a disconnected rambling of unassociated thoughts.

Ganglion: A structure housing a group of nerve cell bodies.

Hallucination: A distortion of a sense, auditory or visual, that occurs in the absence of a true stimulus. The apparent perception of something that is not actually present.

Hemoglobin A1C: A form of hemoglobin that measures the average blood glucose concentration over a three-month period. It is now used to monitor for progression to diabetes and as a measure of effectiveness of diabetes treatment.

Hippocampus: A structure of the brain located in the temporal lobe. It is part of the limbic system and plays important roles in memory, spatial understanding, and emotions.

Homeostasis: The tendency of the body, or any system, to attempt to maintain a balance or equilibrium in its internal environment by regulating variables, even when there are external changes.

Hypothalamus: A structure of the brain located below the thalamus responsible for certain metabolic processes and activities of the nervous system. One of its most important roles is its link of the nervous system to the endocrine system via the pituitary gland. It is responsible for production of many of the body's essential hormones and through that helps to govern many physiologic functions such as sleep, mood, hunger, sex, and temperature regulation, among others.

Illusion: A distortion of the senses that leads one to perceive something incorrectly. An illusion is a misinterpretation of true sensation.

Limbic system: A system in the brain that includes multiple structures, including the hypothalamus, amygdala, hippocampus, and thalamus. It is key in the regulation of our emotions as well as our memory formation. It plays a large role by influencing the endocrine and automatic nervous systems.

Mesocortical pathway: One of the dopaminergic pathways. It connects the ventral tegmentum to the cerebral cortex. It is thought to be underactive in schizophrenia, leading to a decrease in dopamine and negative psychotic symptoms.

Mesolimbic pathway: One of the dopaminergic pathways. It connects the ventral tegmentum to the nucleus accumbens. It is thought to be overactive in schizophrenia, leading to excess dopamine and positive psychotic symptoms.

Negative symptoms: Psychotic symptoms that are associated with a disruption or change to a normal emotion or behavior. The symptoms include inactivity, amotivation, poverty of thought and speech, flattening of affect, and social withdrawal.

Neologism: Refers to a new word. Seen in thought-disordered people who often combine two words or simply create a new word whose meaning is not known to others.

Neurotransmitter: Naturally occurring (in the body) chemicals that transmit information between neurons. They play a major role in shaping daily functions by the information they transmit from nerve to nerve.

Nigrostriatal pathway: One of the dopaminergic pathways. It connects the substantia nigra to the dorsal striatum and is thought to be unaffected by schizophrenia. It is impacted by antipsychotics that lead to a decrease in dopamine here and unwanted movement side effects.

Nucleus accumbens: A part of the brain near the hypothalamus that makes up part of the basal ganglia. It houses dopamine receptors and is part of the mesolimbic pathway. It plays a large role in addiction and processing fear, impulsivity, and motor.

Orthostatic hypotension: Low blood pressure occurring upon moving suddenly from one position to the next, generally from lying to standing or sitting to standing. Known colloquially as a head rush or dizzy spell.

Peripheral nervous system: The part of the nervous system that is made up of the nerves and ganglia outside of the brain and spinal cord.

Phenothiazine: An organic compound that is used in chemical manufacturing as a stabilizer or inhibitor. It has multiple chemical derivatives that have been found to be useful in various fields of medicine, including allergy medicine, psychiatric medications, and antimalarials.

Pituitary gland: The major endocrine gland that is about the size of pea and located as a protrusion off the hypothalamus. It secretes multiple hormones that help control growth, blood pressure, functions of sex organs, the thyroid gland, and metabolism, among other functions.

Positive symptoms: Psychotic symptoms categorized as changes in feelings, behaviors, or thoughts that were not present prior to the illness. They include hallucinations, delusions, thought disorders, and movement disorders like catatonia.

Reliability: A term used in reference to research that refers to the degree in which the test being studied produces consistent results.

Substantia nigra: A structure in the brain located in the midbrain as part of the basal ganglia. There is a high level of dopamine neurons housed here giving it dark color. It is part of the nigrostriatal pathway and can be impacted in movement disorders.

Systemic lupus erythematosus: A chronic inflammatory autoimmune disease that impacts multiple different systems in the body, including skin, muscles and bones, blood, heart, lungs, kidneys, reproductive, and the brain.

Tangentiality: A nonlinear thought pattern in which the conversation drifts from the initial topic and never returns to the central theme. The conversation begins with a relevant response but then digresses or deviates from the initial subject.

Thought disorder: A disorder of cognitive organization that results in disorganized thought. The conversation can appear illogical, lacking in sequence, maybe delusional or bizarre, or maybe severely impoverished. It can be associated with multiple psychiatric disorders but most commonly is associated with schizophrenia.

Toxoplasmosis: A parasitic disease that is usually spread by eating undercooked food, exposure to infected cat feces, or from mother to child during pregnancy. Acutely it causes a flu-like sickness, and those with intact immune systems generally tolerate it well. It can become latent and eventually create cysts in the central nervous system, including the brain, that lead to neuropsychiatric symptoms.

Tuberoinfundibular pathway: One of the dopaminergic pathways. It connects the arcuate nucleus to the pituitary gland. It is thought to be unaffected in schizophrenia. It is impacted by antipsychotics that lead to a decrease in dopamine here and can lead to an unwanted increase in prolactin.

Validity: A term used in reference to research that refers to how well a test actually measures what it is attempting to measure.

Ventral tegmentum: A group of neurons located near the midline of the midbrain with many dopaminergic cell bodies. It is origin of the dopamine cell bodies of the mesocorticolimbic system and plays a large role in addiction, motivation, and cognition.

Bibliography

American Psychiatric Association. *DSM 5*. Arlington, VA: American Psychiatric Association, 2013.

"Antipsychotic medication use in nursing facility residents." *American Society of Consultant Pharmacists,* 2016. https://www.ascp.com/articles/antipsychotic -medication-use-nursing-facility-residents.

"AstraZeneca to pay $520M settlement in Seroquel lawsuit." *Genetic Engineering & Biotechnology News*, 2010. http://www.genengnews.com/gen-news-highlights/ astrazeneca-to-pay-520m-settlement-in-seroquel-lawsuit/78565333/.

Barrio, Pablo, Albert Batalla, Pere Castellví, Diego Hidalgo, Marta García, Ana Ortiz, Iria Grande, Alexandre Pons, and Eduard Parellada. "Effectiveness of long-acting injectable risperidone versus oral antipsychotics in the treatment of recent-onset schizophrenia: A case–control study." *International Clinical Psychopharmacology* 28, no. 4 (2013): 164–170.

Beaulieu, Jean-Martin, and Raul R. Gainetdinov. "The physiology, signaling, and pharmacology of dopamine receptors." *Pharmacological Reviews* 63, no. 1 (2011): 182–217.

Bloche, Maxwell Gregg. "Uruguay's military physicians: Cogs in a system of state terror." *JAMA* 255, no. 20 (1986): 2788–2793.

Bonnie, Richard J. "Political abuse of psychiatry in the Soviet Union and in China: Complexities and controversies." *Journal of the American Academy of Psychiatry and the Law Online* 30, no. 1 (2002): 136–144.

Carpenter, William T., and James I. Koenig. "The evolution of drug development in schizophrenia: Past issues and future opportunities." *Neuropsychopharmacology* 33, no. 9 (2008): 2061–2079.

Centers for Medicare and Medicaid Services. "Action plan for (further improvement of) nursing home quality." Retrieved November 10 (2008).

Centers for Medicare and Medicaid Services. "Description of antipsychotic medication quality measures on nursing home compare." 2012.

Christian, Robert, Lissette Saavedra, Bradley N. Gaynes, Brian Sheitman, Roberta C. M. Wines, Daniel E. Jonas, Meera Viswanathan, Alan R. Ellis, Carol Woodell, and Timothy S. Carey. "Tables of FDA-approved indications for first- and second-generation antipsychotics." 2012.

Daemmrich, Arthur, and M. E. Browden. "A rising drug industry." *Chemical & Engineering News* 83, no. 25 (2005): 28–42.

"Eli Lilly to pay $1.5B in drug marketing case." *Money.Cnn.Com,* January 15, 2009. http://money.cnn.com/2009/01/15/news/companies/eli_lilly/.

Elkes, Joel, and Charmian Elkes. "Effect of chlorpromazine on the behaviour of chronically overactive psychotic patients." *British Medical Journal* 2, no. 4887 (1954): 560.

Englisch, Susanne, and Mathias Zink. "Treatment-resistant schizophrenia: Evidence-based strategies." *Mens sana monographs* 10, no. 1 (2012): 20.

Ford, Elizabeth B., and Merrill Rotter. *Landmark Cases in Forensic Psychiatry*. Oxford, United Kingdom: Oxford University Press, 2014.

Fosnight, S. "Delirium in the elderly." *Geriatrics* (2011): 73–96.

Frankenburg, Frances R. "History of the development of antipsychotic medication." *Psychiatric Clinics of North America* (1994).

Freudenreich, Oliver. "Differential diagnosis of psychotic symptoms: Medical mimics." *Psychiatric Times* 27, no. 12 (2010): 56–61.

Hirschfeld, Robert M. A., Charles L. Bowden, Michael J. Gitlin, Paul E. Keck, Roy H. Perlis, Trisha Suppes, Michael E. Thase, and Karen D. Wagner. "Practice guideline for the treatment of patients with bipolar disorder (revision)." *Focus* 1, no. 1 (2003): 64–110.

Jaffe, Ina, and Robert Benincasa. "Old and overmedicated: The real drug problem in nursing homes." *National Public Radio* (2014).

Kay, Stanley R., Lewis A. Opler, and Jean-Pierre Lindenmayer. "Reliability and validity of the positive and negative syndrome scale for schizophrenics." *Psychiatry Research* 23, no. 1 (1988): 99–110.

King, David J. "Atypical antipsychotics and the negative symptoms of schizophrenia." 1998.

Lawler, Brian. "Antipsychotic drugs: Technologies and global markets." *Bccresearch.Com,* June 2010. http://www.bccresearch.com/market-research/pharmaceuticals/antipsychotic-drugs-markets-phm063a.html.

Lehman, Anthony F., Jeffrey A. Lieberman, Lisa B. Dixon, Thomas H. McGlashan, Alexander L. Miller, Diana O. Perkins, Julie Kreyenbuhl et al. "Practice guideline for the treatment of patients with schizophrenia." *American Journal of Psychiatry* 161, no. 2 supplement (2004): 18–20.

Lickey, Marvin E., Barbara Gordon, and M. E. Planas Domingo. *Medicamentos Para Las Enfermedades Mentales: Una Revolución en Psiquiatría*. Labor, 1990.

Lieberman, Jeffrey A., T. Scott Stroup, Joseph P. McEvoy, Marvin S. Swartz, Robert A. Rosenheck, Diana O. Perkins, Richard S. E. Keefe et al. "Effectiveness of antipsychotic drugs in patients with chronic schizophrenia." *New England Journal of Medicine* 353, no. 12 (2005): 1209–1223.

López-Muñoz, Francisco, Cecilio Alamo, Eduardo Cuenca, Winston W. Shen, Patrick Clervoy, and Gabriel Rubio. "History of the discovery and clinical introduction of chlorpromazine." *Annals of Clinical Psychiatry* 17, no. 3 (2005): 113–135.

Marder, S., and T. Stroup. "Pharmacotherapy for schizophrenia: Side effect management." *UpToDate.com* 9, no. 15 (2013): 11.

Meltzer, Herbert Y. "The role of serotonin in schizophrenia and the place of serotonin-dopamine antagonist antipsychotics." *Journal of Clinical Psychopharmacology* 15, no. 1, supplement 1 (February 1995): 2S–3S.

"Mental health myths and facts." *MentalHealth.gov*, 2016. https://www.mental health.gov/basics/myths-facts/.

Merritt, Kate, Philip McGuire, and Alice Egerton. "Relationship between glutamate dysfunction and symptoms and cognitive function in psychosis." *Neuropsychopharmacology of Psychosis: Relation of Brain Signals, Cognition and Chemistry.* November 26 (2013).

Mitchell, Alex J., Davy Vancampfort, Amber De Herdt, Weiping Yu, and Marc De Hert. "Is the prevalence of metabolic syndrome and metabolic abnormalities increased in early schizophrenia? A comparative meta-analysis of first episode, untreated and treated patients." *Schizophrenia bulletin* 39, no. 2 (2013): 295–305.

Möller, Hans-Jürgen. "Management of the negative symptoms of schizophrenia." *CNS Drugs* 17, no. 11 (2003): 793–823.

Moncrieff, Joanna. *The Bitterest Pills: The Troubling Story of Antipsychotic Drugs.* Springer, 2013.

Montejo, Angel L., Laura Montejo, and Felipe Navarro-Cremades. "Sexual side-effects of antidepressant and antipsychotic drugs." *Current Opinion in Psychiatry* 28, no. 6 (2015): 418–423.

Nielsen, Jimmi, Corina Young, Petru Ifteni, Taishiro Kishimoto, Yu-Tao Xiang, Peter F. J. Schulte, Christoph U. Correll, and David Taylor. "Worldwide differences in regulations of clozapine use." *CNS Drugs* 30, no. 2 (2016): 149–161.

Olfson, Mark, Marissa King, and Michael Schoenbaum. "Treatment of young people with antipsychotic medications in the United States." *JAMA Psychiatry* 72, no. 9 (2015): 867–874.

Raedler, T. J., F. P. Bymaster, R. Tandon, David Copolov, and Brian Dean. "Towards a muscarinic hypothesis of schizophrenia." *Molecular Psychiatry* 12, no. 3 (2007): 232–246.

Schatzberg, Alan F., and Charles DeBattista. *Manual of Clinical Psychopharmacology.* American Psychiatric Association Publising, 2015.

Seida, Jennifer C., Janine R. Schouten, Shima S. Mousavi, Michele Hamm, Amy Beaith, Ben Vandermeer, Donna M. Dryden, Khrista Boylan, Amanda S.

Newton, and Normand Carrey. "First-and second-generation antipsychotics for children and young adults." 2012.

Seo, Dongju, Christopher J. Patrick, and Patrick J. Kennealy. "Role of serotonin and dopamine system interactions in the neurobiology of impulsive aggression and its comorbidity with other clinical disorders." *Aggression and Violent Behavior* 13, no. 5 (2008): 383–395.

Shen, Winston W. "A history of antipsychotic drug development." *Comprehensive Psychiatry* 40, no. 6 (1999): 407–414.

Shulman, Matisyahu, Avraham Miller, Jason Misher, and Aleksey Tentler. "Managing cardiovascular disease risk in patients treated with antipsychotics: A multidisciplinary approach." *Journal of Multidisciplinary Healthcare* 7 (2014): 489.

Stahl, Stephen M. *Stahl's Essential Psychopharmacology: Neuroscientific Basis and Practical Applications.* New York: Cambridge University Press, 2013.

Stahl, Stephen. *Stahl's Essential Psychopharmacology: Prescriber's Guide*, 5th ed. New York: Cambridge University Press, 2014.

Stead, Latha, S. Matthew Stead, and Matthew S. Kaufman. *First Aid for the Psychiatry Clerkship.* McGraw Hill Professional, 2005.

Thomas, Katie. "J.&J. fined $1.2 billion in drug case." *The New York Times,* April 11, 2012.

Thomas, Katie. "J.&J. to pay $2.2 billion in Risperdal settlement." *The New York Times,* November 4, 2013.

Toda, Mitsuru, and Anissa Abi-Dargham. "Dopamine hypothesis of schizophrenia: Making sense of it all." *Current Psychiatry Reports* 9, no. 4 (2007): 329–336.

"Top antipsychotic drugs in the United States based on revenue in 2011–2012 (in million U.S. dollars)." *Statista,* 2016. http://www.statista.com/statistics/242480/sales-of-antipsychotic-drugs-in-the-us/.

Tse, Lurdes, Alasdair M Barr, Vanessa Scarapicchia, and Fidel Vila-Rodriguez. "Neuroleptic malignant syndrome: A review from a clinically oriented perspective." *Current Neuropharmacology* 13, no. 3 (2015): 395–406.

U.S. Food and Drug Administration. "How drugs are developed and approved." http://www.fda.gov/Drugs/DevelopmentApprovalProcess/HowDrugsareDeveloped andApproved (2012).

"What is metabolic syndrome?" *Nhlbi.Nih.Gov,* 2016. http://www.nhlbi.nih.gov/health/health-topics/topics/ms.

Woolley, D. W. "Serotonin in mental disorders." In *Hormones, Brain Function, and Behavior: Proceeding of a Conference on Neuroendocrinology, Held at Arden House, Harriman, New York, 1956,* p. 127. Academic Press, 1957.

Young, Su Ling, Mark Taylor, and Stephen M. Lawrie. " 'First do no harm': A systematic review of the prevalence and management of antipsychotic adverse effects." *Journal of Psychopharmacology* 29, no. 4 (2015): 353–362.

Index

Abnormal involuntary movement scale
(AIMS), 130, 165–166
Acetylcholine, 91, 200–201
Acute intermittent porphyria, 16–17
American Psychiatric Association,
158–159, 208
Anticholinergic medication, 30, 128
Antihistamines, 26, 29–30, 58, 204
Antipsychotic use in special
populations: children, 119–120,
186–188; elderly, 117–119,
185–186; elderly with agitation and
psychosis, 118; pregnancy, 120–121
Anxiety disorders and use of
antipsychotics, 212–213
Arcuate nucleus, 79
Aripiprazole (Abilify), 48–50, 102,
155–157
Assisted outpatient treatment (AOT),
182–184
AstraZeneca, settlement, 157
Attention-deficit/hyperactivity disorder
(ADHD), 7
Atypical antipsychotics, mechanism of
action, 85–86, 90
Autism spectrum disorder, diagnosis,
course and treatment, 113–114

Basal ganglia, 80, 105, 125
Bipolar disorder, diagnosis, course and
treatment, 111–113, 211
Brief psychotic disorder, diagnosis,
course and treatment, 110

Center for drug evaluation and research,
branch of FDA, 153
Centers for Medicare and Medicaid
services, regulation of antipsychotic
use in nursing homes, 159–160
Central nervous system, 64, 74
Cerebral Cortex, 75, 79
Chlorpromazine (Thorazine),
26–27, 30–33, 59
Clinical Antipsychotic Trials of
Intervention Effectiveness (CATIE),
67, 100–101, 105
Clozapine, 42–45, 66–68, 105–107,
161–163; regulation of, 163–165;
use in treatment resistant
psychosis, 195
China, 184–185
Cold water baths, 54

Deinstitutionalization, 62–63,
170–171

Delirium, causes and treatment, 115–116

Delusional disorder, diagnosis, course and treatment, 109–110

Diagnostic and Statistical Manual of Mental Disorders, 20

Disruptive mood dysregulation disorder, 13

Dopamine: pathways and functions, 78–80; receptor types, 80–81; synthesis, 77–78

Dopamine hypothesis of schizophrenia, 28, 82–83

Dorsal striatum, 80

Efficacy of antipsychotics, 103–104

Electrocardiogram (EKG), 136

Electroconvulsive therapy (ECT), 55

Exorcism, 25

Fluphenazine (Prolixin), 39–41

Food and drug administration (FDA): mission, 153; regulation of drug production, 153–154; relationship to pharmaceutical industry, 151–152, 155–157, 159

Freeman, Walter, 56–57

Frontal lobe, function of, 74–75

Gage, Phineas, 75

Gamma-aminobutyric acid (GABA), 91, 202–203

Genetics, use in the treatment of psychotic disorders, 199–200

Glutamate, 91, 201–202

Haloperidol (Haldol), 37–39, 66

Hippocrates, 25

Histamine, 91, 204

HIV, 116

Homelessness and mental illness, 173

Human Genome Project, 199

Hypothalamus, 80–81

Impulsive aggression, causes and treatment of, 101–103

Incarceration and mental illness, 173–174

Indications for antipsychotic use: nonpsychotic disorders, 110–114; primary psychotic disorders, 107–110; psychotic disorders secondary to a medical condition, 115–117

Insulin shock treatment, 54–55

Intermittent explosive disorder, 13

Intranasal antipsychotics, 210–211

Janssen Pharmaceuticals, development and production of Risperdal and Invega, 154–155

Johnson and Johnson, development and production of Risperdal and Invega, 154–155; settlement, 157

Kendra's Law, 182–183

King George III of England, 14–15

Laborit, Henri-Marie, 58–59

Limbic system, 83

Lobes of the brain: frontal, 56, 74–75, 79; occipital, 74–75; parietal, 74–75; temporal, 74–75

Lobotomy, 26, 55–57

Long-acting injectables, current and future, 205–208

Lupus, 116

Lysergic acid diethylamide (LSD), 87–90

Major depressive disorder and use of antipsychotics, 212

Major depressive disorder with psychotic features, diagnosis, course and treatment, 110–111

Malaria, 116

Mesocortical pathway, 79, 84

Mesolimbic pathway, 79, 84

Metabolic monitoring, 166–167
Moniz, Antonio Egas, 56

National Institute of Mental
  Health, 7, 100, 212
Negative psychotic symptoms, 20, 82,
  99–101, 194–195
Neuroleptics, history of term, 19
Neurosyphilis, 116
Neurotransmitters, definition of, 76
Nigrostriatal pathway, 80, 84
Nucleus accumbens, 79, 81

Occipital lobe, function of, 74–76
"Off label" medication use, 13
Olanzapine (Zyprexa), 101, 196
Oppositional defiant disorder, 13
Otsuka, development and production of
  Abilify and Rexulti, 155–157
Oxytocin, 91, 204–205

Parietal lobe, function of, 74–75
Parkinson's Disease,
  48, 64, 69, 125–127
Pathophysiology of psychotic
  disorders, 198
Peripheral nervous system, 74
Perphenazine (Trilafon), 34–36, 101
Pharmaceutical industry: history of,
  152; relationship to psychiatry,
  158–159
Phenothiazine, 26
Pituitary gland, 80, 138
Positive and negative syndrome scale
  (PANSS), 104
Positive psychotic symptoms: delusions,
  20–22, 94–98; perceptual
  disturbances, 22–23, 94–96, 194;
  thought disorders, 23–25, 94–95,
  98–99, 194
Pregnancy, medication classes, 121
Prior authorization, in regulation of
  antipsychotics, 160–161
Prolactin, 80

Psychosis, definition of, 19
Psychotropic, definition, 19

Quetiapine (Seroquel), 47–48, 212

Rennie v. Klein, 180
Reserpine, 63
Risperidone (Risperdal), 45–46,
  154–155
Rogers v. Commissioner, 180

Schizoaffective disorder, diagnosis,
  course and treatment, 108–109
Schizophrenia: diagnosis, course and
  treatment, 5–6, 107–108; cost of,
  194; treatment-resistant, 44, 88,
  162–164, 195–197
Secondary psychosis, causes, 116
Serotonin: future use, 203–204;
  pathways and functions, 87;
  synthesis, 86–87
Serotonin hypothesis of psychosis,
  87–89
Side effects: acute dystonia, 127–128;
  akathisia, 128; clozapine-induced
  agranulocytosis, 106, 142–144;
  clozapine-induced myocarditis,
  144–145; clozapine-induced seizures,
  145; constipation, 138; excessive salivation, 145–146; extrapyramidal
  symptoms (EPS), 124; hyperprolactinemia, 139; metabolic syndrome,
  131–135; neuroleptic-induced parkinsonism, 125–126; neuroleptic
  malignant syndrome, 140–141; QT
  prolongation, 135–138; sedation,
  130–131; sexual side effects,
  139–140; tardive dyskinesia, 65,
  128–130
Soviet Union, 184
State v. Perry, 181
Substance-induced psychotic disorder,
  diagnosis, course and treatment, 114
Substantia nigra, 80–81, 125

Temporal lobe, function of, 74–75
Thioridazine (Mellaril), 33–34
Toxoplasmosis, 116
Treatment over objection, 178–184
Tuberoinfundibular pathway, 79–80, 84
Typical antipsychotics: high potency,
   36–42; low potency, 29–34;
   mechanism of action, 28–29, 84–85;
   mid potency, 34–36

Uruguay, 185

Ventral tegmentum, 79
Violence and mental illness,
   190–192

Wyatt v. Stickney, 70

Ziprasidone (Geodon), 101

About the Authors

JEFFREY KERNER, MD, is an attending psychiatrist at Montefiore Medical Center, Bronx, New York. He is forensic coordinator of the inpatient unit at MMC-Wakefield and assistant professor of psychiatry and behavioral sciences at Albert Einstein College of Medicine. Kerner is the author of "Corporate Greed as an American Evil" in Praeger's *A History of Evil in Popular Culture: What Hannibal Lecter, Stephen King, and Vampires Reveal about America.*

BRIDGET McCOY, MD, is a general adult psychiatry resident at Montefiore Medical Center, Bronx, New York.

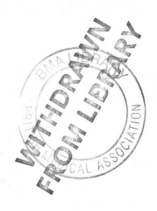